How to Understand and Deal with Health Anxiety

HOW TO UNDERSTAND AND DEAL WITH HEALTH ANXIETY

An Hachette UK Company
www.hachette.co.uk

Vie Books, an imprint of Summersdale Publishers
Part of Octopus Publishing Group Limited
Carmelite House
50 Victoria Embankment
LONDON
EC4Y 0DZ
UK

www.summersdale.com

Printed and bound in Poland

ISBN: 978-1-83799-319-2

Substantial discounts on bulk quantities of Summersdale books are available to corporations, professional associations and other organizations. For details contact general enquiries: telephone: +44 (0) 1243 771107 or email: enquiries@summersdale.com.

How to Understand and Deal with Health Anxiety

EVERYTHING YOU NEED TO KNOW TO MANAGE HEALTH ANXIETY

Katy Georgiou

DISCLAIMER

Neither the author nor the publisher can be held responsible for any injury, loss or claim – be it health, financial or otherwise – arising out of the use, or misuse, of the suggestions made herein. This book is not intended as a substitute for the medical advice of a doctor or physician. If you are experiencing problems with your physical or mental health, it is always best to follow the advice of a medical professional.

Contents

Introduction   6

CHAPTER 1:   8
Understanding Health Anxiety

CHAPTER 2:   50
How to Manage Health Anxiety

Conclusion   149

Resources   150

About the Author   153

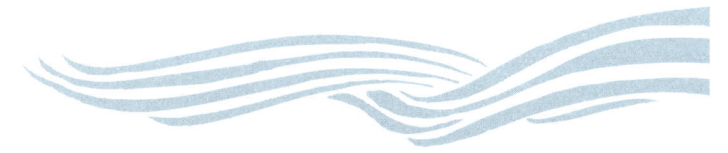

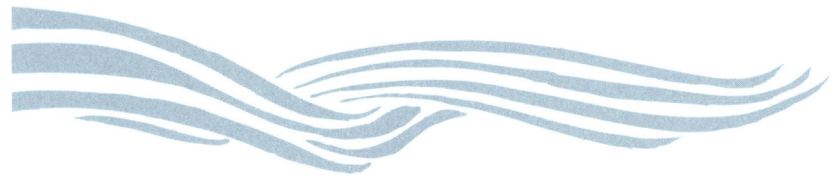

Introduction

Anxiety is a natural part of being alive, and if we never felt it, we simply wouldn't be human. But there is a difference between common anxiety, in times of change and stress, which affects every single one of us, and clinical anxiety, which can feel scary to tackle alone and can affect your quality of life.

There are different categories of clinical anxiety, which the *Diagnostic and Statistical Manual of Mental Health Disorders* (*DSM-5-TR*) divides into obsessive-compulsive disorder (OCD), phobia, panic disorder, social anxiety, generalized anxiety and illness anxiety disorder. Health anxiety is on a scale and fits into the bracket of illness anxiety disorder. It has many overlaps with OCD (intrusive thoughts about illness and associated compulsive behaviours), however, the thoughts are specifically about health and disease. Symptoms are usually experienced physically, mentally and emotionally and often involve worrying about your health to the point of feeling unable to function.

In the following pages, you'll learn how to recognize health anxiety and deal with it if you think you are experiencing it. In the first chapter, you'll learn what health anxiety is, what causes it, and how to spot symptoms and triggers in yourself. The second chapter will help you to manage these symptoms, offering physical exercises, practical tips and techniques. You'll also learn how to talk to a loved one about what's worrying you and how to access formal therapeutic and holistic support if you need it. Throughout the book, you'll have a chance to fill in blank sections in your down time, with the help of guided exercises and prompts to support you.

This book is a trustworthy resource to return to any time you feel yourself wobbling. It will equip you with different options to try, so you can see what works for you. The tips will help you to manage your health anxiety, but try not to put pressure on yourself to find a quick fix. Remember that health anxiety cannot necessarily be cured completely, and there isn't one perfect solution. Everyone is different, and if you're really struggling, there'll be pages here that signpost you to professional support. There's also a handy resource section that you can use, with a list of websites and charities you can reach out to. So, take comfort in this book, sit back and start your journey towards a better peace of mind.

CHAPTER 1
Understanding Health Anxiety

Anxiety is nature's way of alerting us to danger and keeping us going. Without it, we'd likely get little done, though in large doses it can overwhelm us. If someone runs up behind you, it would be normal to jump and for your heart rate to increase. But problems arise if symptoms like this are happening without clear reason, or if they feel out of proportion to what's going on.

In the case of health anxiety, these symptoms are specifically linked to thoughts and fears around your physical or mental health. You might have fears around developing a serious disease, such as cancer, which you ruminate on even if you have no symptoms. You may start interpreting common ailments, such as a headache, as signs of something more sinister. These thoughts become all-consuming and difficult to shake off. This, in turn, can raise your heart rate, increase tension in your body and heighten your fear that you're going to make yourself ill, leading to more worry in a loop that can leave you feeling exhausted, ashamed, withdrawn and hopeless.

If this is happening to you, remember that it's more common than you think and that there is a way out of this, even if it doesn't feel like it right now. This chapter will help you better understand if health anxiety is affecting you, and if so, how it may manifest itself, giving you the science, triggers and causes behind it.

LAYING IT ALL OUT

In the next few pages, you'll learn in more detail about what health anxiety is, some of the science behind it, who it affects, how to spot it and what causes it. You'll discover how to identify your personal triggers, what health anxiety can feel like in your body and the different ways it can manifest itself.

You'll also find some fill-in pages to help you keep track of your feelings and work out if health anxiety might be what you're experiencing. These come with supportive writing prompts to guide you and encourage you to reflect on why you think you have health anxiety.

You'll learn to track sensations in your body, anxious thought patterns, the times of day you have them and what's triggering them.

Anxiety is a natural response to uncertainty and change. But when it starts to consume your everyday life and leaves you feeling like you can't cope, that's where this book will help.

Identifying health anxiety

Anxiety is felt in the body physically but comes with thoughts and fears that you can't let go of. Sometimes the physical symptoms happen first, triggering these thoughts, or vice versa. If this process happens enough times, you might pre-empt your symptoms, which brings them on and intensifies the fear.

"WHAT IF" THOUGHTS

You might start to "worry about your worry", which can feel scary and develop into more "what if" thoughts, such as "What if I never get over this?" or "What if there's something seriously wrong with me?" This situation can lead to panic or feeling hopeless.

FIXING ON A THEME

With health anxiety, it's common for one particular theme around health to play on your mind continually, such as getting ill, dying, going to hospital, fearing a misdiagnosis and double-checking symptoms.

CHECKING AND AVOIDING

You might seek constant reassurance from others, which only lasts a short time, or you might try to control your worries, such as not eating in restaurants for fear of food poisoning. This can restrict your life and have knock-on effects, like losing too much weight, which can be exhausting and difficult to explain to others who don't appear to understand. It's important to know that these experiences are very common. Professionals understand and there is a lot of help available.

What causes health anxiety?

Health anxiety will usually show up during a big life change or a period of stress, but it can sometimes feel as if it's happening out of the blue.

Stresses and changes aren't always obvious but can creep up on you. Perhaps you've been doing fine for a while, but recently things have built up and, like a jar of water filled to the top, one tiny drop leads to an overspill.

Take a moment to imagine your life jar. What are the big and small events that have happened in your life over the last few months? It can help to write these as a list on a piece of paper and divide it up into "big things" and "little things". Big things might include a recent bereavement, an accident, a break-up, moving abroad or changing jobs.

Alternatively, they could be traumatic events like an assault or even near misses, such as putting your foot out as a motorcycle goes past, that you find yourself still thinking about later. Smaller things might include deadlines or an argument with a friend. Remember, these don't even have to be bad things — even happy, positive life events can be stressful, such as a proposal, having a baby or a promotion. Write them all down.

Have I got health anxiety?

If you picked up this book because you think you might have health anxiety, use the following two exercises to clear up doubts about your experiences. In the fill-in section below, explore the reasons why you think you are suffering from health anxiety. Allow yourself to write as freely as possible without trying to get it right. You can keep this for yourself or show it to a trusted friend or loved one and get them to give you some feedback.

....

....

....

....

....

....

....

....

....

....

....

Place a tick next to every statement below that rings true for you. If you tick a lot of them, health anxiety might be something you are struggling with. Do not use this exercise to substitute an actual diagnosis. Instead, make an appointment with a doctor.

☐ I am convinced I've got a serious illness.

☐ Health-related news items plague my thoughts daily.

☐ I worry that I'm worrying too much about my health.

☐ Anytime I see or feel a change in my body, I panic.

☐ I fear I am going to catch something, and I try to avoid it.

☐ If I knew how to stop worrying, I would, but I feel like it controls me.

☐ Nothing quells my urge to check symptoms.

☐ I cannot watch films or TV shows that show hospitals, anyone ill or dying.

☐ I have stopped eating certain types of food in case I get ill.

☐ I am scared to go to the doctor in case they confirm my fear.

☐ My doctor has done tests but I am sure they missed something.

☐ I struggle to trust reassurances over my health.

☐ I panic myself so much I feel sick, which raises my fears more.

☐ I avoid certain routes, places or people in case something triggers a panic about my health.

How seeds of anxiety lie dormant and what prompts them to sprout

The films and TV shows we watch and the materials we read about can really affect us, sometimes unconsciously. They sit heavy with us in the background while we're getting on with our lives but bubble up to the surface, usually in moments of change.

Sensational headlines, breaking news reports and trending media topics are powerful and designed to stir us into feelings or action. Every once in a while, something will crop up in the news that really sticks with us. Maybe it's because it taps into something in our world we can relate to, or because it is so unusual, the idea of it happening to us feels terrifying. When this type of news is around a health-related theme, we can develop health anxiety or have health anxiety from the past reignite, especially if the timing of what we're reading or seeing coincides with a time in life when we're feeling vulnerable.

With health anxiety, it is common to absorb details of news reports and fear them happening to you. You might start taking steps to stop this occurring or turn to friends for reassurance. This can happen in the moment or there can be a delayed effect. You might notice, for example, that a health-related film or a news report you remember really affecting you when you were younger has resurfaced as a theme for you later in life and has developed into health anxiety.

Covid-19 is a recent example of how global health news reports affected us on a mass scale. Similar health reports in the past have included hand, foot and mouth disease, Ebola, Bovine Spongiform Encephalopathy (BSE) in the case of the United Kingdom, and in the 1980s, AIDS and HIV. Depending on your age, you might have memories of these. Notice if there are patterns in the things you worry about that are connected to things you watched and read about in your past.

Brainstorm the big news stories you remember from your lifetime. See if they tally up with major events that occurred in your own life or moments when you were blue or out of sorts. Jot down any connections and keep referring to them as you navigate the rest of the book. You might surprise yourself with some powerful insights you never realized before.

....

....

....

....

....

....

....

....

....

....

....

....

How health anxiety shows up

PANIC ATTACKS

A panic attack is the sudden onset of a feeling of terror. It comes along with lots of physical symptoms, like shallow breathing, clammy hands, a racing heart and even fainting. Sometimes, the experience feels so intense you might think you're having a heart attack or dying. You're not, but it can feel frightening. When you have health anxiety, a worry can grow into a panic attack slowly, while at other times, you might suddenly panic at the idea that what you're going through is never going to leave you. If you have lots of panic attacks, you might start to fear having more, which can trigger more panic.

RUMINATING

You might fear having a serious illness or worry that you'll develop one. Your worries might be focused on a specific theme, such as cancer or dying young. This might be because of something you've seen or watched, or an experience you've had, such as a long stay in hospital, family members falling ill or a period of your own illness that triggered a phobia about it happening again. It is common for worries to build on top of each other so that you start worrying about the very fact you are worrying. You may try to think your way out of these loops, only to find that the more you think about the thoughts or try to shut them out, the more intense they become.

A FEELING OF DOOM

Even when you're not panicking or dwelling on specific thoughts, it's common to feel a sense of dread in your body that sits with you for most of the day. This may ebb and flow at specific times, and you might notice a pattern to when it comes and goes. It can be helpful to keep a diary of the times of day this happens and anything you did (such as what you ate or drank, the people you spoke to or what you were doing) just beforehand.

"What if" thoughts: A classic hallmark of anxiety is a thought process that always begins with "What if... ?" Here are some examples — can you relate to any of them?

- "What if I never get over this and end up in a hospital ward?"
- "What if the doctor missed something serious?"
- "What if it's a tumour?"
- "What if there's no exit to escape if I need to?"
- "I know they checked everything last month, but what if it is different this time round?"

"This time" thoughts

Even if you have been through many rounds of the cycle before, it can feel brand new each time it happens. You might be saying to yourself: "This time, it is different." When you catch yourself saying "this time", that is a classic feature of health anxiety.

This is the last way you want to feel. If only you knew how to stop, you would. However, not knowing makes it worse and may leave you feeling shame. "This time" thoughts can also lead you to look for reassurance from people who have already reassured you.

Try to remember that this is not something you can snap out of. Health anxiety can feel like it has a life of its own and it requires someone who understands how it works to coach and support you. The good news is, with practice, it *is* possible to learn techniques to help yourself.

If you are reading this book because you are a friend, partner or family member supporting someone you think might have health anxiety, you might be the person always being consulted for reassurance. This can feel upsetting, as you want to do your best. Show your friend or partner this book or read Chapter 2 for ways you can access support yourself.

Examine your beliefs

Anxiety is difficult enough, but when we are layering untrue beliefs on top of it, it can feel much worse. Look at the statements below and see what they stir in you. Use the space beneath the sentences to write your own statements that are unique to you. This will allow you to pinpoint any unhelpful beliefs, as well as examine what drives your judgements and where they might have come from.

I should not be feeling this way; I have nothing to worry about in life.

Other people have it worse than me; I should not complain.

I need to just snap out of it.

Only weak people feel like this.

There is no hope for me.

I am scared I will be like this forever.

I am scared that even if I am not ill, I will make myself ill from this.

I am afraid that I am going to push my friends, family or partner away.

I am a bad person.

....

....

....

....

....

Why you're doubtful

Health anxiety can feel like your mind is constantly freewheeling. Partly, this is a natural response to uncertainty: trying to make certain the things that are unknowable and that we cannot control. This might be likely for you if you are used to routine, are high-achieving, strive for perfection, worry what people think of you and like to make a good impression.

YOUR RELATIONSHIP TO AUTHORITY

Anxiety comes hand in hand with self-doubt. When you feel unable to trust your own logic, experts and authority figures become the closest route to a definitive answer. However, no matter how expert, there is always a door left ajar for error. An anxious person will always look for that loophole. If a doctor says there is a 1-in-10-million chance of you having a disease, you'll likely fear that you are that 1-in-10-million exception. When you are suffering with any kind of anxiety disorder, it is being able to bear uncertainty, live with doubt and nurture trust that can feel like the biggest struggle of all.

PAUSE HERE

Hopefully by the time you get to the end of this chapter, you'll feel a little more equipped, empowered, in control, and less alone. For now, just take a moment to breathe and give yourself a mental hug. When you are ready, keep reading.

Who health anxiety affects

Before you took a pause, you read that being a high achiever, someone who feels safe with routine or worries about what others think can be factors in health anxiety. There are some other factors, such as if it runs in the family, if you have a history of another anxiety disorder, or if you witnessed somebody close to you going through a bout of ill health. These all count.

The next few pages go through possible causes for health anxiety, the triggers and what makes you susceptible. Remember that this is just a rough map. Health anxiety can affect anybody, at any age and the reason for it does not always matter. It can even be unhelpful sometimes to look for a reason if there isn't an obvious one. But if the traits do relate to you, this can help it make sense.

If you do not have health anxiety but you picked up this book because you are worried about a person you know, some signs to look out for are:

- Turning down invitations to go out.
- Insisting on taking a different route somewhere.
- Skipping class or not turning up for work.
- Changes to eating patterns.
- Noticeable weight loss or weight gain.
- Asking you similar questions over and over.

Connecting the dots

Health anxiety can be linked to high levels of stress, including big changes happening in your life that set your mind and body into a kind of flux. Sometimes, the effect of these changes on our emotional lives can happen outside of our own awareness: because of that, we miss the telltale signs that something is out of whack. If this goes on for a long time, our bodies start kicking back and giving us powerful clues. These might be physical symptoms, such as heart palpitations, rashes or colds, which lead to the thought spirals and intrusive thoughts we explored earlier.

On page 25, you will find an activity page to help you reflect and brainstorm some of the stresses and life changes you're going through at the moment. This will help you to take stock of any symptoms that you're experiencing, which might paint a picture of why you are going through such a tough emotional time right now.

If anxiety already runs in your family, you strive for excellence at work, home and in studies, you pride yourself on being reliable and are prone to feelings of guilt, then it makes sense that in moments of big change, those shifting sands can really challenge you. That's because, in moments of transition, the future is not clear. Even if you are excited, our bodies are creatures of habit and want to get back to their biological state of equilibrium as fast as possible. In this space of limbo, there is no way for your feelings to truly land, and that's a heavy load for your mind and body to carry.

In short bursts your body will handle this, but in time it will start to act out and fill in the vacuum. It can be helpful to imagine an earthquake: some areas are more prone to them, but they aren't happening all the time. Under certain conditions, the tectonic plates shift, which shakes the ground and brings up foundations. This is usually the moment when the freewheeling symptoms and intrusive thoughts start.

Witnessing trauma

If you lost someone close to you to disease or illness at some point in your life, if you witnessed someone die or had a brush with illness yourself, this can be a huge factor in why your anxiety is health-specific. This is especially the case if what you went through was traumatic and unexpected, and you did not have much time to think before acting.

Sometimes, in moments of trauma and acute stress, our bodies do not have time to register what is happening as we have no choice but to attend to the emergency and stay safe. But because of how human bodies and brains are wired, the sober reality of what happened and your own mortality can hit you later. This can throw you into uncertainty and fear around how fleeting life can be, which might be short-lived or more enduring.

BRUSHES WITH LIFE AND DEATH

Traumatic incidents do not have to show up in such obvious ways. Sometimes, a close call such as almost putting your foot out of a car door as a motorbike comes past can have a similar effect on you.

On the next page, you'll have a chance to identify any near misses or traumatic events in your life and an opportunity to consider if you think your life history could be a factor.

Reflect on your life history

Warning: if you find that you're spending a lot of time trying to "search" for trauma in your past, do not do this exercise.

This exercise will get you thinking about aspects of the past that might play a role in how you're feeling today. It is not always the case that health anxiety works this way, but if trauma has been in your life, it can be useful to consider it as part of the picture.

TASK 1

Plot a quick timeline of your life on some paper with key dates and events. You can write it as a list, draw images or even voice it out loud to a trusted friend.

TASK 2

Look at your paper and see if anything jumps out. If you trust someone else to look at it, they might to spot obvious things that you did not notice.

Some pieces of the puzzle might start to make sense, but don't worry if they don't. This isn't a test, and not everyone will fit the same template.

A summary so far

As you have worked your way this far into the book, you will have absorbed a lot of information. It is a lot to take in in one go. Allow yourself some breathing space to let what you have learned sink in. To help remind you, here is a summary of what we have explored so far:

SYMPTOMS

- **Physical symptoms**: heart palpitations, stomach churning, feeling sick or dizzy, shallow breathing, hyperventilating, fatigue and exhaustion.
- **Emotional symptoms**: feeling fed up, out of control, afraid, hopeless, depressed, desperate, sad, lonely, angry and nervous.
- **Thought patterns**: you worry all the time about your health, being ill, dying, missing an underlying condition, doctors being wrong or test results being wrong.
- **Behaviours**: you scan your body and check symptoms online constantly. You hone in on a specific illness and do everything you can to avoid it. You visit the doctor, pharmacy or clinics frequently or avoid appointments completely, as well as scenarios that might expose you to illness, like eating out. You doubt yourself, double check and seek reassurance that never reassures. You say "what if" and "this time" constantly, and you picture yourself ill, in hospital or something happening to you.

TRIGGERS

- Scenes on TV, such as hospital dramas that show people ill, in hospital, being sick, dying of illness.
- News coverage of epidemics and pandemics (such as the Covid-19 pandemic).
- A family member falling ill, a stressful life event or a near-death experience.

All of these can be factors that trigger your initial bout of health anxiety or bouts that follow. It can also feel completely random, as if there is no trigger at all.

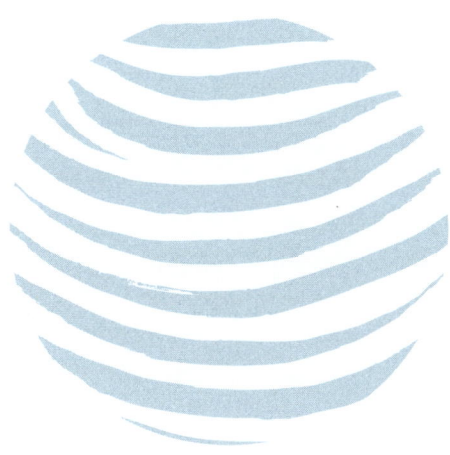

Getting clearer

By now, you might have a clearer idea of whether or not what you're going through is health anxiety, something else or one part of a bigger picture. In these pages you'll start to learn a bit more about risk factors and the science behind it all.

RISK FACTORS

- **Your genes**: according to the National Alliance on Mental Illness (NAMI), health anxiety, like other psychological disorders, can run in your family. Research has shown that genetics, when combined with a stressful event, situation or environment, increase the risk of health anxiety.
- **Your physical health**: some medical conditions can cause and create feelings of anxiety. These include diabetes, an overactive thyroid and asthma, and any other psychiatric disorders. This is tricky because the crux of health anxiety is that you're worried you have a medical condition, so if a medical condition is creating the anxiety, then you're going to be even more concerned. However, a good doctor will understand how to separate these things. They usually check your medical history first and run tests to rule these aspects out. Once that condition is treated, this would remove the symptoms of anxiety.
- **Your lifestyle and environment**: the way you live, the people around you and your surroundings can all affect your chances of developing health anxiety. If you are highly stressed, experience a traumatic incident, drink a lot of alcohol or take recreational drugs, this can all increase your risk.

Questions to reflect on

Answer "yes" to any question that relates to how you've been feeling over the last few months. Then write down on a scale of 1-10 *how* much it's been affecting you, where 1 is barely at all, and 10 is in every minute of every day.

Question	Yes/No	1-10
Are you convinced or worried that you have a serious illness?		
Any time you experience an unusual sensation or symptom, does this trigger you into a spiral of worry?		
Is it interfering with other areas of your life, e.g. social life, work, friendships, finances?		
Are you constantly researching information about this illness either online, in books, or from consulting doctors and experts?		
Do you still feel worried even when you receive reassurance?		
Are you avoiding situations out of fear of becoming ill?		
Do you have a family history of health anxiety or another similar disorder?		

Exploring a bigger picture

As humans, we're complex, and how our lives play out can be a combination of genes, biology, how we were parented and brought up, the people we met growing up, significant events that happened to us, how our belief systems were conditioned, the phase of life you are in, the current stresses you are under, and your relationships.

This includes your very early childhood development, even when you were a baby. How attuned your caregivers were to you and the moral codes they taught you have a huge impact on your world view. When we get older, we can believe that we're independent in our own thoughts and opinions, but you'll be surprised by just how many of our actions are rooted in beliefs that were instilled in us from a young age by those who influenced us.

Getting a diagnosis

The *DSM-5-TR* refers to health anxiety as illness anxiety disorder. It is a relatively new diagnosis. People can have health anxiety for many years before it gets diagnosed, but it's more common than we realize. Because it can occur alongside other things, trigger or feed into other mental health issues, these separate conditions might be diagnosed before health anxiety.

For example, if you've been having panic attacks because of health anxiety, the panic disorder might be diagnosed before the health anxiety. It's important to know that psychiatrists have a developed understanding of these things and can recognize when there is a bigger picture at play. To be diagnosed, the issue must be affecting your life considerably, and symptoms need to have been there for at least six months. Diagnosis is done through a process of elimination. Organic diseases are ruled out, and then a careful assessment takes place, factoring in your whole history. If you feel you need a psychiatrist, their role will be explained in more detail later in this book.

If you have health anxiety, you're more likely to consult a doctor before thinking of therapy because you won't necessarily be making the connection. It's something that is frequently misdiagnosed, but studies suggest that this is changing because our attitudes to health in general are different, and more people are reporting health concerns to doctors who, in turn, recognize their symptoms as those of health anxiety.

Myths about health anxiety

FALSE: People with health anxiety are only anxious about symptoms they don't have.

TRUE: Having a negative health-related experience in the past can trigger health anxiety.

FALSE: People with health anxiety are hypochondriacs.

TRUE: Hypochondriac is an unhelpful term that shames and stigmatizes a person and prevents their chances of receiving appropriate support.

FALSE: People with health anxiety are just desperate for attention.

TRUE: People with health anxiety often suffer in silence or avoid talking about it. They are mostly desperate *not* to be experiencing it.

FALSE: You must be anxious about your health all the time to have health anxiety.

TRUE: Health anxiety can be a sudden onset (acute), frequent bouts or chronic (there all the time).

FALSE: Health anxiety means you are going mad.

TRUE: There are professionals out there who are trained to understand what is happening to you and know what to do to help.

FALSE: Everyone gets health anxiety if they think they are ill.

TRUE: Health anxiety is not the same as anxiety when awaiting results. For example, if somebody goes to the doctor with a suspected lump and is referred for a biopsy, the person will almost certainly experience anxiety in the run up to the biopsy and awaiting the result – this is not health anxiety, but a common and normal response. Health anxiety is when the anxiety *is* the issue: simply even reading the previous sentence, for example, might be enough for you to worry about needing a biopsy. Check which camp you fall into.

The most recent version of the *DSM-5-TR* removed hypochondriasis as a diagnosis due to the disparaging connotation in its name, though it still remains in the World Health Organization's (WHO) *International Classification of Diseases* (*ICD 11*). The *DSM-5-TR* term is illness anxiety disorder. To be considered as illness anxiety disorder, symptoms must affect your daily life so much that you cannot cope.

The science behind health anxiety

Health anxiety isn't your fault, but it also isn't out of your hands completely. Comprehension of the brain and nervous system can be a really useful first step to understanding how anxiety works. Next you'll get to learn a bit about the basic science of the brain and the role your nervous system plays in it. You'll also get to understand how brain cells communicate and lead to anxiety developing or getting worse. It's by no means the full picture, and the other pieces of the puzzle will be explored too, but it's a good place to begin.

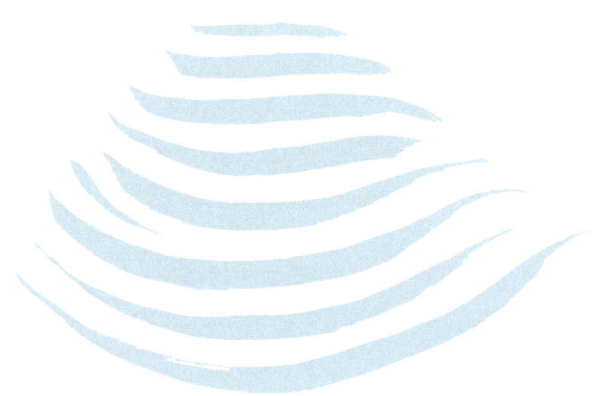

Learned behaviours

Use this page to take stock of some of your beliefs and attitudes. How much are they yours, and how much are they from learned experience?

....

....

....

....

....

....

....

....

....

....

....

....

Neural pathways

A neural pathway is the route your brain takes to send signals from one part of it to another. All along the route are brain cells. These are called neurons, which are the vehicles for these signals to travel through. There are different types of neurons: motor neurons (controlling our muscles), sensory neurons (dealing with our senses) and inter-neurons (connecting the neurons, a bit like hooks that join two trailers together).

The more the signals run along a neural pathway, the stronger it becomes. It would be like walking a well-worn hiking trail. As people up ahead learn which paths to trust, they signal to people behind that it's safe to walk there.

We are born with many of these pathways already formed, but as we live and grow, we develop new ones all the time. A fascinating part of how we're built is that we can actually control which pathways we create or close off. The more we reinforce one pathway, the more it grows, and we can start taking the route out of habit. Quite literally we can change pathways or think new pathways into existence at any time. We can also close off old roads that no longer serve us. The brain is really flexible and able to adapt in this way. Neuroscientists call this neuroplasticity: like plasticine, you can change its shape and which way it goes.

This can be a really hopeful message if you're experiencing health anxiety, because it means that you *can* change or influence your brain. It's just about knowing *how* (Chapter 2 will cover this).

When you've got health anxiety, you've forged a route in your brain that signals run along out of habit. It's not your fault: you weren't to know. The building blocks of what caused that route may have happened when you were too young and being conditioned by what was around you at the time.

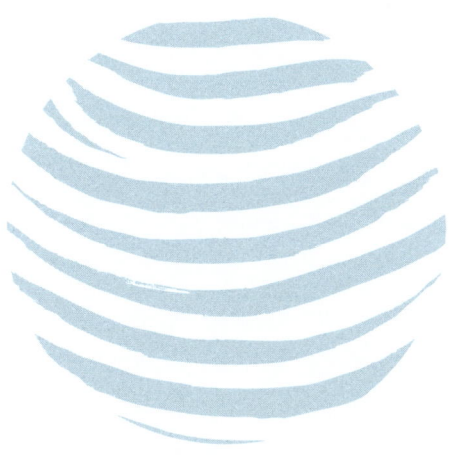

How biology and childhood interact

You might have grown up in a tense environment, which prepped your brain to be extra vigilant, but you might have also just learned to respond to anxiety in the same way your caregivers did or taught you to do, for example, through avoidance rather than tolerating the anxiety. Having health anxiety does not in any way mean that you had a traumatic or frightening childhood. The vast majority of parents and caregivers want the best for their children, but sometimes they accidentally model ways of coping that don't serve you well later in life.

When the brain is dysregulated, or in other words, not fully managed, we can second guess ourselves constantly. If we never learned the skills to cope when younger, why would we know how to do it now?

Use the prompts on the next page to reflect on these things and make some notes.

SOME PROMPTS FOR REFLECTION

How were you parented as a child?

....

....

....

....

Were you trusted to do things by yourself?

....

....

....

....

How did you learn to manage your anxiety?

....

....

....

....

More detail on the brain

Your brain is divided into three parts: your survival brain, emotional brain and thinking brain.

The survival brain deals with your basic body functions that keep you alive and existing, such as heart rate, breathing, movements, temperature and sleep cycles.

The emotional brain (part of the limbic system) deals with everything to do with emotions, feelings and awareness of danger to keep you safe. It's here that things like fear and stress are activated. It also contains a part of the brain called the amygdala, which you can learn about on the next page.

The thinking brain (prefrontal cortex) is the most recent part to have evolved and deals with your relationships, language, imagery, communication and formation of meaning. It is very sensitive to stress.

Within your thinking brain is your hippocampus, where memories are stored. The amygdala attaches emotions to them, while the cortex attaches logic. These parts work together, usually in harmony. When we're anxious, a chain reaction of events is happening via the amygdala or prefrontal cortex.

The amygdala

Your amygdala is like your personal bodyguard that scans for threats and protects you from danger. It raises the alarm when trouble is ahead and helps you to process positive emotions.

This is a wonderful thing as it keeps us safe from harm. When we're doing well, we can trust it to let us know when something's wrong. But when there's an anxiety disorder, it goes haywire. It starts sending us alarm bells at moments when there is no danger, and even if there is, once it has passed, the alarm doesn't stop.

Where we could previously switch off, now we lose trust. We second guess the amygdala. Once this happens, your body is no longer just responding to threat but preparing for a red alert, which, of course, triggers the alert again. Our lives become a cycle of worrying about the fact we're going to worry until, eventually, we worry about the fact we worry so much it becomes tiring.

Many people who experience this might notice a small window of peace at certain moments in the day, such as that moment of waking from sleep. But once your memory kicks in, the tripwire is triggered off again. This can lead to a feeling of physical exhaustion, which, in turn, can leave you feeling hopeless or depressed.

Recognizing those signs in yourself is important as they can escalate. If you're supporting someone going through this, understanding these effects can build a fuller picture of the problem.

Stress responses

When your anxiety feels out of the blue, this is usually a telltale sign that the amygdala is involved. However, when you reflect on what was happening leading up to that anxiety, usually you can identify that you were in a particular place or situation that triggered it.

When the amygdala signals danger, your body prepares to protect itself. This triggers a stress response: anxiety floods the brain with the stress hormones cortisol and adrenaline, which, in turn, alert the amygdala. This affects your rational thinking and conditions your brain to hold negative memories.

TYPES OF STRESS RESPONSE

We have five key stress responses: flight, fight, freeze, flop and friend. These are hard-wired responses to keep us safe, usually connected to how we responded to threat in our very early development.

- **Fight**: where you confront and try to defeat the thing that's overwhelming you.
- **Flight**: where you run away, avoid or retreat to escape danger.
- **Freeze**: where you feel stuck, like a rabbit in headlights, and cannot move. This is usually because escape does not feel like an option, running away would lead to being chased by the danger, or fighting risks harm to yourself.
- **Flop**: where you go "offline" as if you are not there. Your muscles become floppy, you might feel dizzy, faint or, in more extreme cases, dissociate (when your thoughts and feelings disconnect from your body). This usually happens if freezing still isn't enough to stop the threat of harm. It is a very common response to trauma.
- **Friend**: where you move closer to the threat or make friends with it because it is your best chance of staying safe.

Usually, after a stress response is activated, it subsides — but not with health anxiety. This is because the rational part of the brain that usually makes sense of what's happening stays offline. The amygdala stays in emergency mode for longer, triggering more adrenaline and cortisol in the body that, in turn, make the body tense, the heart beat faster, and breathing become quick and shallow. This tenseness can sometimes feel as bad as the fear itself. These symptoms can become mistaken for something more serious, such as a heart attack, which subsequently triggers a panic attack. This is why it's easy to see why you might worry about being ill.

As we have learned, however, the brain adapts and changes continually. You can change what's happening to those chemicals and brain parts towards a happier life: that's a well-researched, biological fact. Knowing this, by itself, can be a huge relief.

Neurotransmitters

All these communications happen through a network of cells called neurons. There are billions of neurons in the brain, each one separated by a little space (synaptic cleft). The signals travelling through this network across these spaces are electrical and chemical impulses called neurotransmitters. Dopamine is an example of a neurotransmitter. It's the one that we commonly describe as "feel-good".

While electrical impulses trigger and help the communication travel from neuron to neuron, it's the neurotransmitters that dictate the flow. Like a tap that gets turned on or off, they alter the flow through the tap so that more or less of it circulates. When the tap is opened, it's to make more of something happen, and when it closes, it's to reduce what's happening and calm you back down. This process of neurotransmission is called synaptic transmission.

WHEN THE FLOW OF COMMUNICATION GOES WRONG

Sometimes, this communication can go wrong: the neurons might produce too much or not enough neurotransmitters (such as dopamine), or some transmitters may get absorbed too quickly or slowly. Occasionally, enzymes (special proteins that speed up chemical reactions in the body) can attack neurons.

The neurotransmitters and hormones involved in anxiety include serotonin, adrenaline and cortisol. For a long time, many professionals believed that absorption of serotonin was a key issue for anxiety, and this led to the use of medication called selective serotonin reuptake inhibitors (SSRIs). Current thinking around medication and anxiety has changed a lot in recent years, as Chapter 2 will explore.

Create a thought diary

A thought diary is used in cognitive behavioural therapy (CBT) (see page 99) to help you recognize patterns of what happened in the lead up to your anxiety spiral. Use the space below to write your thought diary.

Every time you feel anxious, a thought creeps in or you have a panic attack, log the details on this page or in a notebook, stating when and where it happened and the circumstances around it. It can take a few days or weeks, but see if you can spot any patterns, such as the time of day they happened, who you were with and anything you were doing just before, like eating a meal or going on a night out. Once you spot a pattern, your experience should feel a little less random.

....

....

....

....

....

....

....

....

....

Your prefrontal cortex

The amygdala (threat receptor) isn't the only route to anxiety. The prefrontal cortex (thinking brain) has a role to play, and the two play off each other.

While the amygdala is a short circuit to a more instinctive, primitive and emotional place, the prefrontal cortex dwells in thoughts and imagery. It takes the information it's receiving (sights, sounds, ideas, thoughts) and tries to make sense of it for you. When it's functioning properly, it should figure out if something is worth worrying over or not and then report back to the amygdala to dial down the alarm or raise it higher. But sometimes, the prefrontal cortex isn't alert enough, and it doesn't regulate the amygdala. Like one parent not noticing that their child is about to run into the road, while the other acts as if the child has already been knocked over, they are out of sync.

Other times, the thinking brain *is* alert, but it's interpreting things incorrectly. This can happen if there's been a past trauma and a negative memory stored in your hippocampus, which means that your thinking brain is using that information each time that it encounters anything, instead of thinking independently to keep you safe.

This all makes sense when we consider that people can experience health anxiety in two ways. Sometimes the physical symptoms of anxiety happen first. The feelings come from nowhere, randomly and irrationally, and without any logic or apparent reason. But in other moments, it's the thoughts and images that come first, which lead you to interpret those thoughts, which then trigger the physical and emotional feelings.

Sometimes one can lead into another, or you can start out in the first camp, but get to a point where you're pre-empting the anxiety, which takes you to the second camp and vice versa. See if you can identify in your thought diary on page 45 which type of anxiety you were having and when.

When your body gives you signs of anxiety out of the blue, it's your amygdala playing up. But when it happens the other way round, or in other words, the intrusive thoughts and images come first, that's usually a telltale sign that your prefrontal cortex is at play.

People experience their anxiety differently, some more in one way than the other, and sometimes a combination of the two. The longer the anxiety goes on, the more likely both will happen.

Taking stock

Understanding the anatomy and biology of the brain, as you've just done, can go a long way in providing you with some relief around what you are going through. In clinical settings, this kind of information-giving is termed "psycho-education". Psycho-education is often used by professionals as part of their approach to treatment. For some, this learning can be enough to resolve the issue by itself. If that's happened to you, take comfort in the power of this and return to this book in moments when you feel yourself doubting or worrying. It can help make sense of things, but it can also help support you when you come to further treatment and recovery if you need it.

If it doesn't feel quite enough, that's okay. Sometimes it takes somebody experienced to be able to see what is going on for you and guide you to redirect your thought loop so that it goes on a different path. While eventually you can start to do this for yourself, for now, free yourself of that burden and simply surround yourself with people who understand that the thought loop is not deliberate. If they don't, try not to tackle their beliefs by yourself: show them this book.

As you move into the next chapter of the book, you will start to learn how to tackle your health anxiety and access help if you need it.

Draw your life jar

Near the start of this chapter, on page 11, you were invited to think about your life jar. Use this space below to draw it and notice how you feel.

CHAPTER 2
How to Manage Health Anxiety

Now you have understood what health anxiety is, how it shows up and what your triggers are, this next chapter will give you tools, support and guidance for managing it. This section includes practical and physical tips to try at home and well-known, researched strategies from the world of therapy, medical and alternative health. It will also provide information as to who and where to turn to if you need more formal support.

If you're supporting someone with health anxiety, there will be information for you too. As you work your way through this section, remember that these are general guides and tips that are not intended to replace any professional advice you have been given. It is important not to self-diagnose, and if at any point you feel your anxiety is impacting your day-to-day life, seek out the professional support provided in the resources section (page 150).

The first part of this chapter will guide you through supportive practical exercises, self-help, self-care and well-being tips that you will be able to practise any time by yourself to help you manage your symptoms. If you are ready to speak to someone about how you are feeling, this chapter guides you through how to reach out for help and the different kinds of support available to you. Examples of this include talking to family and friends, seeking out support from charities or your local community, and accessing more professional, structured treatment and support in the form of psychotherapy, medication and holistic health.

There will be sections to help you identify what kind of support you need, explore the differences between treatment and support, and reflect on what you've learned so far through guided fill-in pages. The final pages will talk you through what to do if you are the person supporting someone with health anxiety.

Whether you are reading this because you or someone you know is going through a hard time right now, a list of resources at the end of the book will signpost you to a range of books, charities and organizations worldwide. The hope is that you feel more equipped and armed with a range of information to help you take the next steps forward.

Helping yourself

The idea of this self-help section is that you should be taken on a journey from panic to recovery — beginning with a set of tips, techniques and exercises to help in moments of emergency. The initial exercises focus on helping you self-regulate and getting back to feelings of safety. The tips that follow aim to support you when you are not panicking but feel anxious and want to stop the anxiety developing.

These exercises work to help you divert and channel your thoughts elsewhere and recreate neural pathways to achieve a more relaxed state. Finally, you'll work through exercises that help increase your resilience and your capacity to cope. This will mean that you are less likely to feel anxious in the first place, or when you do, it doesn't impact you as much.

Inhale, exhale

When we are anxious, we can forget to breathe, take shallow breaths or hold our breath. Focusing on your breathing and getting yourself back into rhythm will gently shift your attention away from your thoughts and increase oxygen to the brain, which helps to calm you down. Use the following exercises to get you out of a panic state.

- Place your feet flat on the ground, close your eyes and draw in a deep breath as if you're drawing it from the ground through your feet and into your legs. Keep breathing it up to your upper body. Hold for five seconds, then breathe out, imagining your breath leaving your body through your arms and fingertips. Repeat the process.
- Trace the shape of your hand with a finger. Breathe in as you trace your finger upwards, then breathe out as you trace down. Not only does this regulate your breathing, but contact with your skin helps to keep you in the present.

Ground yourself

Contacting the ground is your first defence if your anxiety is turning into panic. As soon as you feel your heart racing, do your deep breathing as described on the previous page and place your feet flat on the ground. Alternatively, sit on the floor cross-legged or lie down flat.

You can ground in a number of ways. Walking barefoot can give you an extra sensation that connects you with your sense of touch. If you are at home wearing socks or shoes, try taking these off. Really feel the temperature or texture of the floor or carpet. Walking on grass, in mud or on a sandy beach are also options.

If you are outside or in the garden, touching and holding plants can really help to keep you "earthed". Hold some soil in your hands and smell it. Studies suggest that soil contains a microbiome that elevates our mood when we become exposed to it. Watering plants also helps.

Alternatively, look upwards and notice three things can you see, hear, smell, taste and touch. Pick out colours in the room and different kinds of light. The point here is that your senses are your best and easiest route back to feeling calm as they take you out of your head and root you back into the present.

Now that you have learned some basic grounding and breathing techniques to support you with the physical symptoms of panic, the next set of pages will help you to come back into the "now" when you are going down a rabbit hole of thought loops.

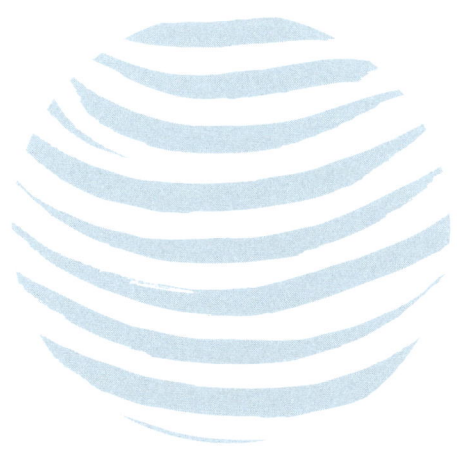

"What if" vs "what is"

On page 10, you read about "what if" thoughts, which are the telltale signs that your issue in a moment of worry about your health is anxiety, not the thing you fear.

This exercise will help you tackle those "what ifs". It can be an especially helpful technique for quashing the pathway to imagining the worst, something some therapists call "catastrophizing".

When you catch yourself saying "what if", change it to "what is" and notice what is *actually* true right now. Often, this is a far cry from what we were depicting in our minds.

STEP 1

When you hear yourself saying "what if", remind yourself this is a sure marker of anxiety, not health.

STEP 2

Change "what if" to "what is".

For example:

What if: "What if I end up in A&E needing an operation?"
What is: "What is happening: I am lying in my bed in my pyjamas with an eye mask on."

What if: "What if that food I just swallowed gets stuck in my throat and I choke?"
What is: "What is happening is I am breathing and talking to my friends."

Avoid catastrophizing

A common technique used in CBT is cognitive restructuring. This helps you to examine your own thoughts and correct your pathway of thinking. In a CBT session, you would work on something like this with a practitioner, but you can do it on your own, too.

Below is a typical form you might get to see when using this CBT technique – give it a try.

1. What are you worried about?

....

2. How likely is it that your worry will come true? Give some examples of past experiences or any other evidence you have to support your answer.

....

....

3. If your worry comes true, what is the worst that will happen?

....

4. If your worry comes true, what is most likely to happen?

....

5. If your worry comes true, what are the chances that you will be okay in a week, a month or a year?

....

Watch yourself

When you're panicking, thinking your way out of it isn't easy. Here are some variations on the "what is" exercise to get you back into the now when self-talk isn't enough. The power of these is that they do not require much thinking, yet they short-circuit any escalation. Think of them as the "watch yourself" techniques, where you observe yourself from an outside perspective.

THE OBJECT TECHNIQUE

When you are anxious, focus on an object in your room. Imagine yourself from the object's point of view. What are you doing with your face, your feet, your hands? See how many details you can draw out from this, such as fidgeting, for example. The idea is that you come to recognize telltale signs of what your body is doing before and during anxiety, and in time, you will read your body in a better way.

THE MIRROR TECHNIQUE

Stand in front of a mirror and stare at your reflection. This can be a powerful way to confront yourself and move away from negative thoughts. Make it your go-to action any time you feel a pang of anxiety. Breathe onto the mirror and look at the condensation. Write "I'm okay," in it. Not only do you get to use the power of touch here, but the next time you pass the mirror, you will be reminded that you got yourself out of a panic: if you did it once, you can do it again. Keep a compact mirror in your bag for moments when you are out.

THE WINDOW TECHNIQUE

When we are suffering from feelings of doom, we can picture all sorts of scenarios in our minds that haven't happened but that we're convinced are going to. In those moments, it can feel like we're already in them or that those things are actually happening. A quick way out of this is to imagine yourself peering through your own window, looking at yourself. What do you see? Usually, it is just you standing in a room, perhaps frowning, but none of those awful things you pictured are truly happening. This can be a helpful reminder that you are safe. It may even make you laugh, which will give you a boost.

THE REAL TIME TECHNIQUE

We can get so caught up in our heads, we can forget what's real, right now, around us. Take a step back from whatever is happening and say the obvious, out loud: "I'm in my room, on a chair, looking at my computer." This can be a sobering way to come back to the present.

Rechannel your thoughts

These exercises rechannel thoughts to help you feel less anxious. Try them out when you are feeling a little tense before panic sets in. For best results, make them part of your routine practice.

The physical act of setting your thoughts to paper can change how you feel about them. Many people do this through journalling. There are many ways to journal — see what draws your attention in this list:

- **Gratitude journalling**: write down everything you are grateful for.
- **Dream journalling**: jot down what you dreamt about. Pick out details from the dream and try writing it out from the perspective of something or someone else who was there.
- **Unsent letter**: to an old partner, someone you lost, your unborn child, a parent, etc.
- **One line a day**: write whatever line comes into your mind.
- **Travel journalling**: document your location or where you might want to visit.
- **Morning pages**: write whatever you like, but always first thing in the morning.
- **Art journalling**: use pictures instead of words.
- **Vision board**: create a physical collage of your future life with images and colours you collect through the day. Look at the board every day and step into that world.

Set aside time for journalling each day and make it a routine. This creates "me time" to channel thoughts in a productive way. On the next page is a fill-in activity for you to practise journalling right now.

My journal for today

Picking a theme from the previous page, use this space below to practise journalling something. Allow in whatever thoughts come and don't overthink it.

....

....

....

....

....

....

....

....

....

....

....

....

Make a scene with visualization

When you feel yourself getting caught in a thought loop, positive visual imagery can help to transport your mind elsewhere and focus on something different, changing how your body feels.

Here are a few suggestions:

Picture a calming scene or somewhere you want to be. This might be a beach, forest, sunset, or a situation like receiving an award or hearing the speeches on your wedding day. Close your eyes and imagine yourself in this place. Notice what the temperature is like. Envelope yourself in that feeling and notice the effect on you. Gently turn your attention to the smells around you and take in a deep breath. Pick out a detail of this scene: the sea, a tree or the sky.

Picture yourself in the future doing something you love. Where are you and who are you with? How are you speaking with them and what about? Take in what that feels like. This technique can help you clarify your goals and give a feeling of long-term hope.

If there was a time in your life when you were not anxious, close your eyes and take yourself there. Notice how this makes you feel. This can be helpful to return to if you want a reminder that life wasn't always like it is now and that it can change again. See if you can spot any clues in that moment: is there anything you can incorporate into your current life?

The buffer techniques

Next is a set of tips to help you buffer your anxiety ahead of time. Think of it like a "future you" who is standing up ahead and looking out for you. You will thank yourself down the line. You can call these the "buffer techniques".

LOCATE YOUR SUPPORT

Support is a way to stop you feeling isolated. It doesn't mean that it gets rid of the problem, but it bolsters you so that, when life gets really tough, it is a little easier to cope with. Support can come in different forms: people, places, things or activities. When you are panicking, it can be so easy to forget what these things are in the moment, so take a minute or two now to reflect on all the different kinds of support you have at your disposal. It might feel like there isn't much, but the more you think about it, the more will come.

The fill-in activity on page 65 will give you some prompts to help you brainstorm your support network. When you find yourself wobbling, just look at the list and you'll have a pre-prepared menu of options to turn to in an instant.

People, places, things, activities

On the next page, jot down the people, places, things and activities in your life that you find supportive. Don't overthink it. If you are stuck, here are some prompts to help you along:

PEOPLE

- Who are the people in your life who are good listeners?
- Who are the people in your life who always seem to know the right thing to say?
- Who do you trust to respect your privacy and confidentiality?

PLACES

- Is there somewhere in your home that helps you to feel calm?
- Is there a café or restaurant that you love going to?
- What are the parks and green spaces that you like visiting?

THINGS

- What smells and perfumes do you love?
- What kinds of textures do you like?
- Do you have pets?

ACTIVITIES

- Name something you do that brings you out of your head and relaxes you: it could be taking a shower, cooking, taking the dog for a walk or doing a food shop. Be as creative or instinctive as you like. It's your book, so do it your way.

When we're in moments of anxiety and panic, it can be difficult to sift through all this information in the moment. That's why having a piece of paper like this to turn to quickly can send us to the right support.

People	Places
Things	**Activities**

The sandwich technique

The sandwich technique lessens the impact of something stressful by sandwiching it between two supportive things that help you cope better. The more you reduce or cushion your stress (if the stress cannot be removed), the more you keep your baseline state calm and regulated.

Anytime you foresee stressful situations, choose a go-to act to do beforehand, then launch into another act when the stressful situation ends. For example, maybe you are dreading a business meeting in the morning. Before work, grab a hot chocolate from your favourite café or put on a necklace with sentimental value that you can hold. Once the meeting is over, email your closest friend for some relief or arrange to go to the cinema after work.

The first supportive act helps build your resilience before the meeting, while having something to look forward to afterwards makes the meeting less important. If you can increase these micro supports so that your stressful event is not the only important thing about your day, it lessens the impact on you.

Remember that stressful situations can include isolated events or they can be enduring situations, such as a dying parent, a break-up or moving abroad. They do not have to be negative either: getting married or having a baby might feel exciting but fraught with tension. If you are in an enduring stressful scenario such as a divorce, then cushion each "mini" stress with the sandwich technique, and then do something supportive again when each day is over.

More prompts for support

Make a list below each prompt. Take some time to think and research what is out there. Doing the work now and consulting the list when you need it will also buffer you.

Podcasts, books, TV shows and films I love:

....

....

Lectures I can go to about health anxiety:

....

....

Clinical trials on health anxiety I can volunteer for:

....

....

Songs and albums I love:

....

....

Hobbies I would be happy to try:

....

....

Make a mixtape

Music impacts our autonomic nervous system (heart rate) and limbic system (emotions), so make a playlist or mixtape that helps take you from one emotional feeling to another. Research indicates that it is a good idea to begin with a song that matches how you feel first, before gradually taking you to a more restful state. The scientific term for this is "entrainment", and it is increasingly being used as a tool in healthcare settings to reduce anxiety before or after operations.

Think back to the songs you were listening to at important moments in your life. Recent studies indicate that your memories are most vivid around age 14. Reflect on what was in the music charts at this time or what you personally remember listening to.

Caution: avoid doing this exercise if your teen years involved trauma. Alternatively, pick a different time of life.

You might even wish to write your daily journals while you listen to music or the playlist you have created.

If you play an instrument, this can be a grounding way to help you work through anxiety. Consider playing a piece that matches your anxiety state, and imagine taking yourself, through the playing, into a more relaxed state.

Your instrument might include your voice. It does not matter whether you sing well or not, just sing it out. There are also options to join choirs or music for well-being groups.

When your heart is beating fast, try playing a song with low beats per minute (BPM). Music therapy research shows that our heartbeat matches the BPM of the song we are listening to, so a low BPM should help to regulate you. If you love live music and can go to a live concert, research demonstrates that the communal aspect of this helps your heartbeat to sync with the crowd. Research also shows that we hear music in the womb: if you are able to learn what your biological mother was listening to at this stage of her pregnancy, try listening along. This is believed to take us back to soothing feelings.

You can cope

A variation of the "what is" experiment on page 56 is "I will cope".

Sometimes, what fuels health anxiety is being so afraid of illness that we try to do everything in our power to prevent it. But human nature copes much better when it is allowed to move forwards and adapt to a situation rather than avoid it. Most things that happen are not the things you were worrying about. It is very unlikely that your health-related fear will happen.

But rather than fighting it, consider this:

If your biggest fear happened, you would cope.

How did this thought just make you feel?

....

....

....

....

....

....

....

....

The previous exercise may have helped you, but if it did not, read through the questions below. If you have a therapist already, you might want to do this exercise with them. If you don't, you could try it with a friend.

QUESTIONS TO CONSIDER

- Do you believe you could cope if your fear happened?
- What do you picture happening if you couldn't?
- Get a closer look at that picture: can you draw out any details from it? For example, who is with you, where are you, what are the consequences?
- What *could* you do in this situation if it happened?

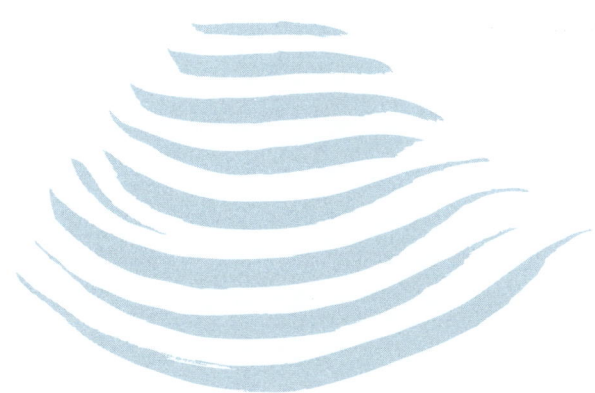

Your physical health

The next few pages will continue looking at your body and health. Emotional and physical health are interlinked. Anything you do to keep your body working and functioning well will have a knock-on effect for how well you cope with your emotions and feelings. Of course, it's easier said than done, but simple changes to your routine and lifestyle can make a huge difference, such as staying hydrated, reducing caffeine intake, moving more, changing how you eat and ensuring you have the right nutrients, vitamins and minerals. The next few pages will guide you through how to make these lifestyle changes.

DRINKING WATER

Cross-sectional studies from *World Journal of Psychiatry* show that there are links between drinking plain water and symptoms of anxiety reducing. Try to aim for six to eight cups of water a day and reduce any caffeine you might be drinking. Caffeine is more likely to increase heart palpitations and make your anxiety worse.

Eat differently

Anxiety can make you want to do things to cope, alleviate feelings of tension or establish control. This can often be through food — either through restricting it, avoiding it or swallowing our feelings with it. Certain foods and snacks have a texture, crunch or taste to them that temporarily alleviate tension in your body. While this can feel comforting in the moment, a long-term increase or decrease in calories and lack of the right nutrients will affect how well your body is functioning. This has a knock-on effect of leaving you more on edge and prone to self-blame. It can be a vicious cycle, but there are ways to tackle this.

Try to limit foods like ice cream, biscuits or cake. Foods high in refined sugar make our blood sugar levels spike, increasing cortisol and affecting the ability to manage feelings well. There are naturally sweet alternatives like cinnamon, honey, prunes and other fruits.

Try not to get bogged down with the idea of "good" food and "bad" food. Instead, take an approach to food as simply "nutritious". Some food items are essential for your nutrition, while others are nonessential. Try to avoid calorie counting and getting too concerned with every ingredient. Even a simple phrase like "eat some vegetables today" can be enough to make a huge difference.

If you think you're really struggling with your eating and the tips above aren't enough to help you, there are professionals who will understand how health anxiety and eating co-exist. Start by visiting your doctor and they may refer you on to specialists.

Move around

It's easy to get stressed when thinking about exercise, and finding the motivation when we're anxious can be difficult. If that sounds like you, just remind yourself to simply move around often. This can be dancing to a song you love, walking around the room, jumping on the spot, stretching or even just shifting position. The idea is to be as fluid as possible, reducing the amount of time you're sitting or standing still.

Once you've got into the groove of making movement a natural part of your day, start doing movements that get your heart beating a bit more, like going up and down the stairs and jogging on the spot. Aerobic exercise affects your metabolism, heart and how good you feel, reducing the levels of adrenaline and cortisol in your body, which are directly related to anxiety. Studies also show that weight training can help reduce anxiety because of molecular changes in the muscles and brain.

Try keeping a weight near to something you use often, like a kettle. Every time you fill that kettle to make yourself a tea, pick up the weight and lift it up and down for the time it takes the kettle to boil. If you're someone who's already very used to exercise and likes to feel the benefits of it, consider making it even more of a routine in your day. This can include walking, running or taking a class. Sometimes interacting with other people in a group exercise class can help move your mind away from your thoughts and back into present focus. Change your exercise a bit each day to keep yourself focused in the now and not caught up in your head.

Like with eating, try not to feel guilty if you don't manage it. Unless you find it helpful, avoid setting yourself strict goals. Instead, just make movement a natural part of your daily routine, like going to bed or brushing your teeth.

WALK ON

Whether it's a brisk walk or a stroll, getting some fresh air and your blood circulating makes a huge difference. Walking can be a great way to help you make sense of what's going on for you and to untangle problems in your mind, while getting your heart pumping.

Try vitamins

We get vitamins and minerals through a balanced diet. They play a massive role in how our bodies work and making sure those neurons are firing properly.

It is understood that being deficient in B vitamins affects anxiety. The best way to get them is through eating meat, fish and eggs, or leafy greens and beans if you're vegetarian or vegan. If you decide to supplement with vitamins, speak to your pharmacist, who will advise you if it's safe, as some vitamins interact with other drugs you may be taking. It's not good to take too many supplements; they won't necessarily get rid of dietary issues, but they can make you feel more able to cope.

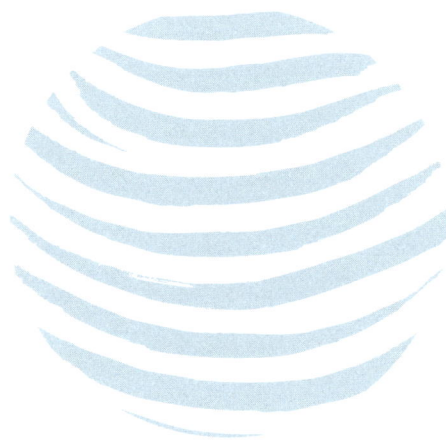

Become your symptom

Below are prompts to stop you fixating on scary bodily sensations and symptoms. Next time you feel something in your body that starts to worry you, imagine being the symptom and speak out from its perspective in the present tense.

For example:

> I am a heart flutter, and I am frantic. I am beating fast and want to get out.
>
> I am trapped here with no escape.
>
> I am a graze, and I am weeping. I am sore and in need of care.

Say these phrases out loud a few times. Notice how they make you feel. Check if the statements you're saying ring true to what you've been feeling. These exercises can be helpful to let you know how you actually feel. Sometimes our bodies send us signals for what we are feeling outside of our awareness.

You don't have to do this exercise alone. If you have a trusted friend, ask if they can take part with you. Get them to repeat back the phrases you make and see how they land on you when you're hearing them back, or ask them to tell you what they feel when they hear you say them. Allow what comes up between you to flow into a bigger, deeper conversation on the topic.

Sleep well

In Chapter 1, you read about how tiring health anxiety can be. Because of the worrying, thinking and checking you are doing, you might flop into bed exhausted, sleep in late, or find it difficult to wake up or stay awake during the day. When you have health anxiety, your sleep patterns can go out of whack. Other times, anxiety might cause you to wake up at intervals or make you afraid of going to bed. The chances are that you already know what poor sleep can do to health, which feeds into fears that you're causing yourself harm which, in turn, keeps you awake. You may interpret your insomnia as a sign that something is wrong.

Everyone has different moments in the day when they feel different levels of anxiety, sometimes higher and sometimes lower. This will influence your sleeping pattern. However, there are things you can do to help you sleep. Not only does sleep help you rest, but it also supports your body to repair, work better and alleviate symptoms of anxiety. Telling someone to rest and sleep with anxiety can feel as futile as saying, "don't worry", but there are tricks you can adopt to help you along.

The Sleep Foundation suggests that quality sleep helps the brain to make sense of emotions. That's between 7 to 9 hours of sleep, but if you're not getting this, don't put too much pressure on yourself. Aim to increase it by an hour or 2 per night for now and work your way up.

Invest in decent bedding, including a supportive mattress, a comfortable pillow and a duvet tog to keep you from feeling too hot or cold. Take naps in the day, try using lavender essential oils or scented products (unless you are pregnant), play music or white noise in the background, avoid caffeine, use meditation apps, go for long walks or a swim, use blackout blinds if you have them, and stop using your phone or computer at least an hour before bed. In fact, you might start to see a link between the hours you choose not to check things online and getting to sleep quicker.

If you have tried all these things and you are still really struggling, consider CBT for insomnia (CBT-I).

Mind and body

YOGA

Yoga is a combination of posture work, breathing, visualization and meditation. There are many different styles of yoga that suit a range of fitness levels: *Ashtanga* (athletic and challenging), *Yin* (slow stretches), *Vinyasa* (poses linked together in flow), *Hatha* (gentle posture and breath work), *Kundalini* (includes chanting), *Lyengar* (precision and alignment), restorative (prolonged postures), hot yoga (in a heated room) and aerial (using fabric hanging from the ceiling to perform movements).

These can be done in your own home with a YouTube video, in a class or on various spiritual retreats. It is a spiritual practice that the WHO recommends due to its mental health benefits for managing anxiety, such as focusing your mind on your breath and away from intrusive thoughts. To get the best results out of yoga, try practising it daily before or after your journalling or just before bed. It supports your mind–body connection at any age.

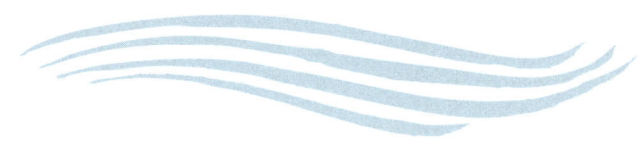

Guided meditations and mindful exercises

Write down how you feel on a scale of 1–10 for each statement, with 10 indicating total agreement and 1 indicating total disagreement:

.... My thoughts are racing.
.... I feel compelled to check my symptoms.
.... I feel anxiety in my body.
.... I want to ask for reassurance.
.... I'm sure I have an illness or disease.
.... I'm afraid of getting ill or having a horrible illness.

After you work your way through this exercise, return to these statements above and jot down how you feel again on a scale of 1–10.

BREATHING EXERCISE

Close your eyes and notice what thoughts come and go in your mind. Breathe deeply in and out, paying attention to your breath.

Start to picture a space between yourself and those thoughts. Open your eyes and focus in on five things you can see, hear, smell, taste or touch.

Your mind will wander during this exercise. It's normal. Each time it happens, stay compassionate to yourself. Name out loud the feelings that have come up and notice where your thoughts have gone, then let them go and bring your focus back to your breathing.

Accept any emotions you are feeling. Imagine they are people in a room you don't know and who'll be leaving soon. Bring your attention back to the here and now, focusing on your breathing and noticing what you can smell, taste, touch or hear.

Meditation

Like yoga, there are different types of meditation. Some are guided and others silent, and all aim to help you feel more at peace. It is research-proven to reduce stress pathways in the brain and affect your emotional regulation.

Note: if you have experienced trauma in your past, research indicates that mindfulness and meditation might not be an appropriate choice for you. Seek advice from a trained professional.

Transcendental: Personalized meditation taught by trained instructors from the Maharishi Foundation, involving sitting with eyes closed for 20 minutes twice per day and meditating with a silent mantra.

Qigong: An ancient Chinese practice that involves harnessing energy in and out of the body through open meridian pathways to help it heal.

Sound bath: This incorporates sound into the meditation through bowls, gongs and other instruments. The vibrations created from the sound help focus the mind.

Zen: From the Zen Buddhist tradition, this involves sitting upright and following the way the breath moves in and out.

Vipassana: An ancient, transformational form of meditation that encourages you to contemplate aspects of human existence to achieve insight and enlightenment.

Mindfulness-based meditation

Mindfulness is one form of meditation rooted in Buddhism, centred around observing what's happening right now without attaching any judgement to it. It is used in CBT to help you cope with your anxious thoughts by encouraging you to observe them like you might a leaf floating down a river and practising letting them "be". The less you attach meaning to them, the less intense they gradually become.

It is understandable to want to stop thinking about difficult things. But trying to get rid of upsetting thoughts can often make us think about them even more. Think of your thoughts and anxiety like a spring: when you try to suppress yourself from having difficult thoughts, they come up with a vengeance, but if you leave a spring alone, it doesn't move. Practising mindfulness helps you to learn how to do this.

Mindfulness-based stress reduction (MBSR) is a formal therapeutic intervention combining yoga and meditation through prescribed courses and daily exercise. You observe your experience as it is happening. This can be combined with CBT to form mindfulness-based CBT (MBCT), which is helpful for anxiety.

Stay mindful

Here are more mindful exercises you can try. Over the next few days, repeat your 1–10 exercise on page 81 with these and see which suit you best. Once you figure it out, set aside regular time to make them part of your routine.

It can be tricky to get the hang of it at first, but if your mind wanders, just gently bring yourself back to the exercise without self-judgement.

Mindful eating: pay attention to the taste, sight and textures of what you're eating, such as the temperature or feel on your tongue.

Mindful exercise: while exercising, focus on the feeling of your body moving. Notice the breeze against your skin and different scents around you.

Mindful colouring: there are many books you can buy now that give you a chance to harness an activity that many of us stopped doing after leaving school. But so much joy can come from that practice. Free yourself to try out different art materials each time. For example, take a crayon and notice how it feels on the page and in your hand compared with a felt tip or a paint brush. Crush bits of crayon into the page and feel it on your skin, or allow yourself some fun to break the rules a bit and flick paint.

Mindful activity: this might be cooking, doing the laundry, washing the dishes, changing the sheets, cleaning the shower or anything else. Pay attention to how things like water feel on your skin, the steam that comes up from your food or the smell of fresh linen.

Mindful meditation: this involves sitting quietly to focus on your breathing, thoughts, sensations in your body or things you can sense around you. Try to bring your attention back to the present if your mind starts to wander. This can be combined with yoga.

Mindful body scan: when your muscles are relaxed, your amygdala receives a message that there's no threat. Notice if you're gritting your teeth or clenching your jaw, and try to relax them. Then close your eyes and drop your shoulders. Make your arm go limp, so that if somebody were to pick it up and let go, it would drop right down again in a thump. Do a quick scan of the rest of your body, relaxing each part as you go.

If you prefer not to do these exercises in your own home space, or if you want company, there are multiple options: courses and classes, private lessons, or guidance through podcasts, apps and YouTube channels. MBCT and MBSR are more structured forms of mindfulness delivered by trained practitioners.

Reaching out

Spotting your symptoms and triggers and learning how to manage them by yourself is already a huge step, but sometimes we need a little help and support along the way from other people in our lives or from professionals who are trained in this area. Over the next few pages you'll learn tips on how to open up to a friend, partner or family member about how you're feeling and explore other avenues of support. It can be scary opening up for the first time, or maybe you've already tried and you didn't get the outcome you'd hoped for – but don't give up. Use these next pages to figure out what you want to say.

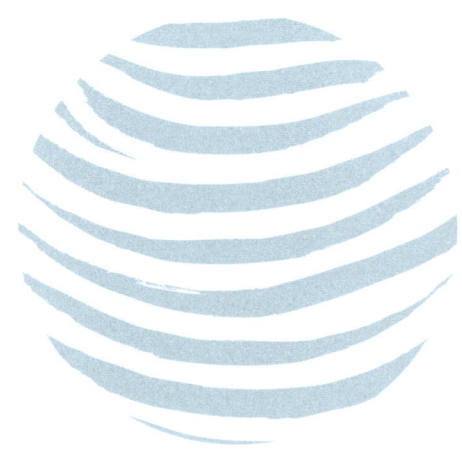

Find community

Going straight to a doctor or professional can feel daunting when you don't know what you're asking for. Charities and helplines can be a safe middle ground as a first step.

Many mental health charities offer free advice and support for what you're going through, such as helplines, drop-in centres, community hub activities, support groups, coffee mornings, networking events and counselling. Some are specific for anxiety while others offer broader support. Charity websites offer a comprehensive list of their services and are also useful resources to tap into for signposting. Do a simple search online and make full use of what's there.

Helplines are usually free and available round the clock. These can be a huge support when offices are closed or nobody else is around, such as in the early hours of the morning when you can't sleep. You'll usually get to speak to a trained volunteer or professional with experience of what you're going through. Some helplines offer practical support, advice and signposting, while others are there simply to give you a space to be heard and explore your feelings when you're struggling.

You'll find a list of these helplines and charities related to health anxiety in the resources section at the end of this book.

Most local communities have communal spaces and activity hubs. These include theatre spaces, community halls, libraries, allotments, churches, mosques, synagogues and other places of worship. Search these for activities that encourage connection and belonging, such as dance classes, choirs, yoga and meditation.

How to turn to a friend

CHOOSING WHO TO TURN TO

Identify who in your life you feel safest talking to. Earlier, on page 65, you outlined all the people, places and things you can turn to for support. Notice who you listed in the people category. Who were the ones who listen well? Are they available?

Flesh out your list. Next to each name, write down how you'd like to contact them — do you want to see them, call them, email them? Don't worry if you can't think of anybody. You'll get to learn other avenues for getting help.

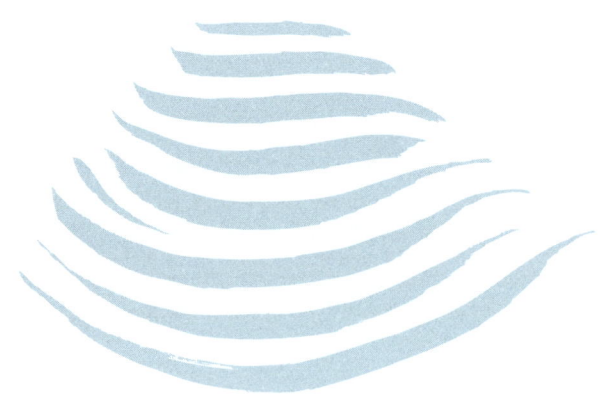

OPENING UP

It can be disheartening when you turn to somebody for support and don't get what you're after. Often people mean well and try their best, but it isn't quite what's needed. Here are some tips for helping you guide someone to giving you the support you're looking for.

- Be clear about what you're after. Is it advice, their opinion, a caring ear or something practical? Before you approach someone else, it can be helpful to be clear with yourself on this first.
- Share your frame of mind.
- Let them know the sort of content they're going to hear.
- Ask them how you'd like them to be with you.
- Give time expectations.
- Do you want to meet, have them call or text?
- Give them notice if you require privacy or will be sharing very personal details.
- Instead of: "Can I call you?" Try: "I'm not coping. Do you have 10 minutes today for me to call you in confidence for advice?" This way, the person can let you know if they can help, and nobody gets hurt.

If you don't get the kind of response you had hoped for, this can feel disheartening. However, there are always ways to turn it around, beginning with letting the person know what you appreciated about their offer and then stating your need.

For example: "I appreciate that you care a lot and you're coming from a good place. Ideally, I'm not looking for advice, but I could really do with a hug."

Professional help

DO YOU WANT TREATMENT OR SUPPORT?

The word treatment is often used to describe professional help. It's worth remembering the following key elements:

Treatment is a process: No two people are the same, and what works for some is different to others. Some people recover quickly — this can be the case if your health anxiety came on recently and suddenly (acute onset) and is tackled quickly with the right approach. For others, it takes a while to figure out what works, while for some, the journey to recovery might feel slower, with peaks and troughs of success. What success means for you might differ from somebody else's perception of it. This may be the case if you've been dealing with health anxiety or bouts of it for a long period of time (chronic health anxiety) and the root is a little more complex.

You're more in control than you realize: It's often the case with health anxiety that you feel at the mercy of it. The effectiveness of the help depends on your relationship to the therapy, how matched it is to your needs and what else you do. Believing that only someone else can relieve you of health anxiety gives it great power.

What does treatment involve?: The word treatment implies that something is broken and needs fixing. It suggests that a professional has the solution to your problem and is trained to administer it to resolve it, a bit like an ointment. When you have something like health anxiety, that idea can — understandably — sound alluring. But be careful. A big part of health anxiety is the belief that you have no power over what is happening to you, and a word like treatment can feed into this. You'll be putting a lot of pressure on yourself for the treatment to work and placing faith in the person giving the treatment. If it doesn't "work", you risk feeling let down, abandoned or that there's no hope. If you have already been down that road, you will know what that feels like.

On the other hand, you might fear the idea of treatment, and this is what's holding you back from reaching out. This might be the case if the thought of somebody "doing" something that you're not in control of makes you feel afraid. A helpful way out of all this is to reframe the word "treatment" as "support".

It can be helpful to work through how you feel about the word "treatment" so that you can feel more informed about what different kinds of help mean and what might work best for you.

Use this fill-in page to reflect for a moment on where you sit with treatment vs support. It's a useful exercise to help you understand how much you feel in control and what's driving those beliefs. It will also help you to streamline a little better the exact help you think you need. For some, it's helpful to think of help as guidance or support.

Medication

Warning: Never take any medication mentioned in this book (or stop taking medication prescribed to you) without consulting your doctor first.

Medication is considered a second-line treatment for illness anxiety disorder (after therapy). We have learned that different neurotransmitters decide how much of a message goes round your brain: like a tap, they increase or stem the flow so that more or less of it goes around. Some medications work to increase the flow of signal and others block them. Some will slow down or block the flow of the neurotransmitters activating the amygdala, and others will switch on the tap for the sleepy prefrontal cortex to wake it up.

There are four main categories of drugs that a medical doctor might prescribe. The below are for reference only — only a professional is qualified to tell you what medication will be helpful for your needs.

- **Selective serotonin reuptake inhibitors (SSRIs)**: these increase serotonin levels in the brain to elevate your mood.
- **Serotonin-norepinephrine reuptake inhibitors (SNRIs)**: these increase serotonin and norepinephrine (noradrenaline).
- **Benzodiazepines**: these are usually a short-term measure to help relieve physical symptoms of anxiety.
- **Tricyclic antidepressants**: these address both your mood and physical symptoms but have strong side effects.

Studies have recognized that people with health anxiety tend to feel safer with therapy than medication. This is often because of the fear of what taking medication will mean for their body.

Who is who

Medication must only ever be prescribed by a medical doctor, including a GP, psychiatrist or hospital doctor. If anybody other than a medical doctor is prescribing you medication, this is a red flag. Below is a quick overview of the different roles within the mental health profession and what they can and can't do. Empower yourself with this knowledge so that you are safer when making decisions about your choice of treatment, support or therapy and so that you know what to ask for.

Neuroscientists: These are specialist scientists who research the brain, diseases of the brain, and develop recommendations for medication and technology. They have a well developed view of how something like health anxiety functions and the biochemistry involved, but they are not therapists or doctors, and you're unlikely to encounter them in a healthcare setting.

Psychiatrists: These are medical doctors who trained in medicine and then specialized in psychiatry. They work mostly in clinical settings, but some have private consultancies. They are qualified to assess you, give you a diagnosis and prescribe medication if they think it necessary. They are also responsible for assessing if somebody is at risk of harm to themselves or others and can make a choice to keep that person safe in a hospital.

Psychotherapists and counsellors: These are the people who deliver therapy. They're the ones you sit in a room with, typically once a week, helping you process or work through your experiences. There are different styles of therapy, which you will learn about later. Psychotherapists and counsellors are highly trained professionals with specialist knowledge, and it is not the same as talking to a friend.

Psychologists: These are social scientists who study the mind. There are different types of psychologists but only clinical, counselling and practitioner psychologists are licensed to give you therapy. They will have a doctorate, followed by a special licence to work with patients. They work closely alongside psychiatrists to conduct assessments and formulate treatment plans, which might include a combination of therapy, medication or other support, and they write up reports for you along the way to track your progress.

The resources section at the back of this book provides more information about regulations, membership bodies and how to find practitioners.

Try therapy

There are many different therapy approaches and each takes a different stance towards working with health anxiety. In Chapter 1, we explored how anxiety could be genetic, medical, or from childhood or current life circumstances. Where you think your health anxiety is rooted will determine which course of therapy style might be better suited to you. It will also depend on your personal preference of how you want to interact with your therapist in the room. For example, some therapists say very little while others talk a lot; some set you goals and homework while others are longer term and free-flowing.

Below and over the next few pages, you'll find an overview of the different therapy styles, followed by an explanation of what that therapy style might look like for you, as well as tips to help you work out which is right for you.

Traditional styles of psychotherapy are usually longer term and focused on building a relationship between you and your therapist. The consistency and routine of weekly sessions are what drive a feeling of safety and, while the process might take longer, it can, for many people, have a cumulative healing effect. Other styles of therapy are shorter and goal-oriented, less concerned with roots and causes, and instead address specific symptoms so that they don't disrupt your life as much. It depends on how much your health anxiety is affecting you right now.

If you feel like you simply cannot cope and your anxiety is getting in the way of your work, or even your ability to hold down a job or be in a relationship, then perhaps a more cognitive behavioural, time-limited approach will be useful to you. Once you reach a point where you're able to cope a bit better, a longer-term style of therapy may then be useful as maintenance or to help you keep exploring. If you're designated a therapist that you don't feel comfortable with, you have a right to stop.

Fact: Research shows that the quality of the relationship you have with your therapist, along with your own desire to be there, are, in fact, the biggest factors in whether the therapy will work for you.

Here are some questions to reflect on if you're thinking about seeking a therapist:

1. Do you want your therapist to direct the conversation first?
2. Do you want someone who will give you answers or who will help you process and explore your feelings?
3. Do you need space to talk out your feelings and prefer your therapist to say very little?
4. Do you want to be set tasks and goals?
5. Do you mind receiving tasks to do between each session?
6. Would you like a chance to go into events of your childhood and past, perhaps exploring how you were brought up or your relationship with the people who raised you?
7. Are you currently undergoing quite a lot of stress and change in your life that you'd like to address in your sessions?
8. Are you more concerned with worries about your future and how to make more meaning in your life?
9. Are you looking to be challenged or for somebody supportive who simply hears you and understands?
10. Are you looking for someone that considers your health anxiety within the context of your sexuality, race or gender identity?

Over the next few pages, you will find information on the different styles of therapy. See if they match with what you have thought about.

Types of therapy

COGNITIVE BEHAVIOURAL THERAPIES (CBT)

These are usually time-limited with a goal in mind and include tasks between sessions. The idea is that how we feel, think and behave is all interlinked. Behavioural therapies focus on changing your behaviour to influence your thoughts and feelings, while cognitive therapies challenge your thoughts which, in turn, affect your feelings and behaviour. Combined CBT works on challenging thoughts and experimenting with new behaviours. This type of therapy is usually quite popular in healthcare settings. Over time, CBT has expanded and informed new approaches.

COGNITIVE BEHAVIOURAL THERAPY FOR HEALTH ANXIETY (CBT-HA)

Many patients with health anxiety might not believe that anxiety is the issue or see it as a problem. As such, a key difference in CBT-HA is that work is done at the very start of the therapy to help you recognize that it's the fear of being ill – rather than being ill itself – that needs addressing. Once that's happened, standard CBT methods continue but are adapted for health anxiety. Your healthcare practitioner will likely do a lot of work with you to help you understand the negative impact of internet browsing (cyberchondria) and to support you out of this cycle of behaviour.

A lot of work will be done to address the part of you that finds loopholes in logic, for example, the idea you will be the one person in a million who has the chance of being ill. You'll be taught how to reduce your compulsion to check and seek reassurance, and you will be directed towards learning to live with uncertainty and doubt. You'll also be asked to keep a diary of your anxiety levels and given a task to avoid checking and monitoring your body on certain days of the week. This might include building up the number of days you're asked not to do it until several days go by without you checking.

Realizing you can change therapist, or stop therapy entirely, whenever you want can be a powerful way to see that you're more in control than you think. This then calms down your anxiety and reduces the intensity for next time. The longer you go without a loop, the less intense the loop becomes and the less frequently it arrives, until it's either gone completely or is at least manageable. You'll learn that there will be moments where it might pop up again, especially in times of stress, but you'll have techniques for how to manage those moments, reduce your overall level of stress and anticipate the moments when you're likely to get stressed. It can be really powerful spotting the signs of change and stress in your life in advance and catching the anxiety out before it arrives.

CBT-HA can be done in person or online. Online can be an option if you know you have health anxiety and feel determined to change things. It can be a little trickier if you think you're likely to give up or sabotage yourself, in which case, having a therapist in person to keep you accountable will be crucial.

Other variations of CBT

ACCEPTANCE AND COMMITMENT THERAPY

Acceptance and commitment therapy (ACT) is considered very relevant to health anxiety. It works by supporting you to accept the idea of death while encouraging you to live fully. It helps you think about what you would like your life to really be about and gets you to question what is really stopping you from achieving that. It helps you to dedicate time to things you love doing, which give you meaning, even if life feels tough. Rather than changing what you're going through, the focus is changing how you relate and respond to these things.

On the next fill-in page, you will explore an ACT technique to help you reduce the amount of time spent checking your medical symptoms and support you in times of uncertainty and doubt.

The ACT technique

The following exercise can be helpful when your anxious thoughts are causing you to doubt facts and the knowledge of medical professionals. It is based on techniques used in ACT. The idea is to know what your core values are and then focus on something that brings you closer to these values every time your mind tries to stick on an anxious thought.

On a scale of 1–10, rank the importance of each value to you (where 1 is not important and 10 is a deal-breaker). Then, on a scale of 1–10, rate each value according to how apparent that value is for you now. Subtract the second number from the first. The numbers you are left with represent how much you are currently deviating from your values in each area of your life. Add up all the scores: subtract the second total from the first total for your overall life deviation score.

Value	Importance	Apparent in your life now	Score
Romance			
Fun			
Work			
Friends			
Parenthood			
Health			
Contribution to the world			
Family			
Spirituality			
Personal development			
TOTALS			

Mindfulness–based CBT

According to the American Psychiatric Association, mindfulness meditation is research-proven to lower the stress response, influence anxiety pathways in the brain, and change the activity in the areas of the brain associated with attention and emotional regulation. MBSR is a formal therapeutic intervention that offers a mix of classes and daily exercises for you to do at home through yoga and meditation.

MBCT combines CBT with MBSR if you're suffering with other common issues alongside your anxiety, such as feeling depressed. Psychologists have found a lot of evidence that shows people who receive MBSR and MBCT are less likely to dwell on worries and can increasingly focus on the here and now.

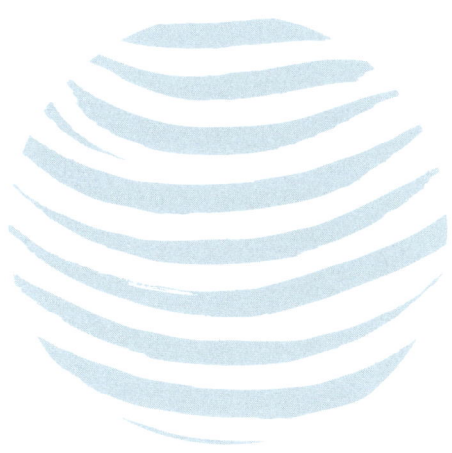

Exposure and response prevention therapy (ERP)

ERP is the most used therapy for obsessions and compulsions. It helps you face your fears and allow thoughts to occur without trying to put them right. It works by exposing you to situations and items that cause a low level of anxiety that you can tolerate. The idea is that, after some time, the anxiety does not get as intense or last as long. You are then exposed to something incrementally more difficult until your ability to cope with anxiety increases.

Your therapist usually takes part in the exercises with you, which can help you to build trust. People report that exposure exercises are not as difficult as they anticipated and that their fears fade away which, in turn, gives them a confidence boost and reduces self-doubt in the future.

PSYCHOANALYTIC AND PSYCHODYNAMIC THERAPIES

These are rooted in the idea that what we're going through is strongly linked to our early developmental years. Your therapist will be very knowledgeable about that but will tend not to say much in the therapy room. Instead, you're given a lot of space to "talk it out". Based on what you say, they may interject to pull out certain words or phrases you've used or to guide you along. They may also offer you an interpretation for what they're hearing, which you might want to consider. The idea is that, through therapy, you re-parent yourself and develop safety and trust.

HUMANISTIC AND EXISTENTIAL THERAPIES

These are rooted in supporting you to find purpose and meaning. They take the approach that your current environment and the context you're living in will impact how you are feeling. Your therapist generally gives you space to lead the direction of your therapy, but through careful listening and back-and-forth dialogue, you're encouraged to reflect and gain insights for yourself.

TRANSPERSONAL THERAPY

This kind of therapy is about aligning your life with your values and higher purpose, which your therapist supports you to uncover.

Compassion–focused therapy

Compassion-focused therapy is a supportive, encouraging, non-shaming approach to addressing your issue by making it clear that the way you respond to life is not something you ever chose. Your therapist supports you to nurture a compassionate, empathetic and reflective voice towards yourself first before inviting you to do anything more complex. Your therapist normalizes your experiences through guided exercises and visualization so you start to build the resources to help you support yourself. It can be helpful if you are prone to feeling guilty or turn to self-criticism and self-blame.

In compassion-focused therapy, compassion-focused imagery is used as a tool for helping you self-soothe. One example of this is picturing your "ideal compassionate self", or in other words, a version of you if you were the most compassionate person ever.

To help you with this:

1. Think about your caregivers and how they supported you growing up, or continue to support you now. Do they do it the way you'd like?
2. If you could tweak it, how would their support look?
3. Can you do this for yourself? Picture yourself this way.
4. Any time you enter a spiral and picture the worst, talk to yourself as this version of you and notice how it feels.

With health anxiety, the process of regulating the threat system is under-developed. It's understood that the endorphins and oxytocin triggered through receiving compassion work together to help soothe you back to a place of calm. Through a process of self-soothing, you help to re-regulate your threat system.

PRACTISE YOUR COMPASSIONATE VOICE

We have just read about nurturing a more compassionate version of yourself through compassion-focused therapy. Imagine being that compassionate person now and write a letter to your current self. This might be a version of you in the future, looking back on yourself now.

Dear..

....

....

....

....

....

....

....

....

....

....

Creative arts psychotherapies

These are different to talking therapies. Instead of talking, you explore your feelings and experiences through music, dance, movement, drama or art. These therapies, especially music therapy, are frequently used in hospital settings and usually for people who find talking difficult, such as people who have had a stroke, a diagnosis of schizophrenia, or are neurodivergent.

Sometimes, you don't need to fit into any of those categories — you just find that expressing yourself comes more easily this way than talking. It can have powerful effects, unlocking feelings and beliefs you were unaware of. Art can also be a safe way to break the rules. Trying to get things "right" all the time can make health anxiety worse. Allow yourself the freedom to colour outside the lines, use colours that do not match, paint with your hands instead of a brush, or put some rags down on the floor so you can flick paint and crush crayons into it. Use the opportunity to see how it feels when you do this. Does it evoke guilt or excitement? Sometimes, it is through "doing" that we can learn who we are. It might take time to build up to all this, especially if avoiding touching things is part of your experience of health anxiety.

Be artful

Art can be a very useful tool in health anxiety to help us access and express emotions that are not always easily put into words. It helps to move your attention away from ruminating thoughts into the present, which helps to regulate the nervous system. Cortisol levels (our main stress hormone) significantly reduce for people who use art forms for stress relief. Try playing around with different creative outlets to see what works for you. As with your journalling, try out various art materials to get a feel for how they work and their different textures: pens, pencils, crayons or paints. If you were to draw your anxiety, what would you draw? Use the space below to try it out.

Group therapy

One of the biggest difficulties you face when experiencing something like health anxiety is the feeling of isolation, as if you're going through it alone. Even if you know there are other people experiencing the same thing, you might not know them, and it can feel lonely having to tackle life with health anxiety by yourself.

There is great power in groups where everybody there is going through the same thing as you. While your stories and backgrounds might differ, simply hearing several other people in the room share experiences that match your own can be very healing. It can be great to talk to people you love, but sometimes, sharing with people you don't know in confidence can help you to feel safe and add a grounding structure and routine to your week. Groups can also be a valuable resource to tap into for trusted information, tips and signposting based on experiences that you can share with each other and report back on.

There are different styles of group support. Formal, structured group therapy happens with the same group of people at the same time and day each week. This is usually time-limited.

Support groups are usually more informal, run by a trained professional or a trained volunteer with lived experience. There are also drop-in groups where you are free to attend a group support when you feel you need it. The people in the group may change each time.

Relationship therapy

Sometimes when you're in a relationship, one or both of you might be feeling left in the dark or feeling guilty about the impact of the health anxiety. This will almost certainly affect your relationship and the way you communicate with each other. Consider relationship counselling with a qualified couples and relationships counsellor, who can give you space to explore how health anxiety is affecting the relationship.

This can sometimes be helpful when everything is said in the open to each other in front of someone trained who can help steer you towards honest and open conversation. There is no shame in this, and it can be a healthy practice to get into.

Fine-tune your therapist

Some people find it important to spend time with a therapist who specializes in a specific theme, such as bereavement, trauma or psychosexuality, or whose specialty is with a specific demographic, such as LGBTQIA+ people, interfaith communities, minority ethnic groups, women or young people. It's helpful to know that such therapists exist, and if this is a factor for you, the resources section at the back of the book will give you more information on where to locate them.

The therapist you choose should still be trained to work with the issue you bring them – in this case, health anxiety. However, they can support you in areas of your life where health anxiety intersects with other issues. For example, if you are a man and you know that your health anxiety was triggered by a traumatic event that resulted in the loss of someone you love, then you may wish to see a bereavement counsellor or trauma-informed therapist who specializes in working with men.

Animal-assisted therapy

This includes visiting farms, zoos or nature reserves and spending time with the animals. Petting and feeding animals can have a very calming effect on the mind. If you don't have access to these things, a visit to a local park to sit by a pond and watch ducks, pigeons and squirrels can ease your anxiety.

Watching animals exist in their own habitats can help you feel connected to a wider world where different living beings live together in harmony. If you like horses, equine-assisted therapy can be helpful, as through assisted interaction with trained horses, you learn to regulate and soothe yourself. Studies have proven that equine-assisted therapy is also very effective if you've experienced trauma.

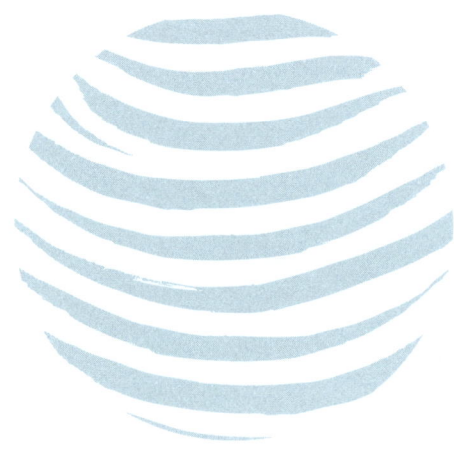

Complementary and alternative therapies

Complementary therapies happen alongside medication and medical treatment. Alternative therapy is instead of medication. Whichever you do, it's always important to discuss this first with a medical doctor to make sure what you're doing is safe. Never abandon something prescribed to you.

The WHO considers complementary medicine a valid form of healthcare to be combined with traditional medicine. Traditional medicine works to maintain your health and prevent illness, drawing on the most up-to-date evidence, knowledge and practice aligned with the beliefs of different cultures around the world. Complementary and alternative medicine is a set of therapies that are not part of a country's main healthcare system but can be used alongside them to alleviate symptoms.

With health anxiety, the idea of complementary or alternative therapies might split you in two ways. They may be alluring because you're afraid of medication side effects, and so they are an option even after medical investigations are closed. Alternatively, they may be scary, in case they don't address the issue you fear is wrong.

They might be a helpful alternative for you if the idea of medication feels too daunting or if your medication is causing lots of side effects. But if you're pregnant, breastfeeding, already on a different medication or you're about to have surgery, then some therapies are less suitable or carry some risk. As such, you should always speak to your doctor first or seek guidance from an experienced practitioner.

If you want to explore this option, then find a practitioner who is registered with a professional body or association to indicate that they meet the right standards of practice. All therapists should be clear about their qualifications, which bodies they belong to and whether they're qualified to work with health anxiety. As with traditional talking therapists, they should be insured. A list of bodies is provided in the resources section at the back of the book.

Get clarity

In the following pages, you will read about the many different types of complementary therapies. However, there are countless more holistic, spiritual, medical, complementary and alternative practices, including homeopathy, shamanic healing, crystal healing, craniosacral therapy, chiropractic technique, the Bowen technique, energy healing and light therapy.

Depending on your cultural, philosophical, religious beliefs, personal attitude, background and history, some may suit you more than others. Use the next fill-in page to reflect on some of your spiritual and religious beliefs to help you decide what kind of practice you'd feel comfortable with.

Take a moment to reflect on your religious, spiritual or cultural beliefs and how you might like that to be respected in a holistic therapy room.

....

....

....

....

....

....

....

....

....

....

....

....

....

....

Massage

There are many kinds of massage, which are outlined below and on the following pages. They almost always involve a practitioner using their hands (or hot stones) to apply pressure and knead certain points of the body. A massage can be grounding and help to relieve the tension you store in your body when you've spent a lot of time feeling anxious. This is because, with anxiety, your body gets tired and tense.

REFLEXOLOGY

This is technically not a massage, but it can seem like one. In reflexology, a reflexologist uses their hands to apply pressure to different points on your feet, which are linked to other parts of your body through your nervous system. It's been found to be effective for aiding sleep.

AROMATHERAPY

In aromatherapy, essential oils extracted from plants are massaged into your skin, with soothing music playing. Earlier, you learned how smell and sound have a rapid impact on the brain. With anxiety, a skilled aromatherapist adapts a combination of oils with the most calming effects, such as lavender oil. You can mix these oils into your own products, or you can find them in candles, but avoid any oils you're allergic to.

INDIAN HEAD MASSAGE

Indian head massage comes from Ayurvedic medicine, which is a philosophy of ancient India promoting health and balance through a mix of products, diet, exercise and lifestyle changes. The National Center for Complementary and Integrative Health (NCCIH) considers Ayurvedic medicine to be one of the world's oldest medical systems.

A skilled practitioner focuses on massaging acupressure points on the head, scalp, face, neck, shoulders and upper back. Usually, you will be sitting upright rather than lying down. Oils are sometimes used, but this is optional. Studies have shown Indian head massage to be helpful in relieving anxiety by stimulating the flow of oxygen in the brain and the parasympathetic nervous system (the part responsible for conserving energy and calming you back down after a fright).

Emotional Freedom Technique

Emotional Freedom Technique (EFT) works a bit like acupuncture but without needles. It involves tapping on points beneath the surface of the skin called "energy meridians". Unlike acupuncture though, you are the one who does the tapping with the guidance of your therapist. For this reason, you might find this approach gives you more of a feeling of control. Along with the tapping, you are encouraged to repeat positive phrases, which results in you feeling more hopeful. Once you have learned this, it is simple to do on your own and can be used to treat fears, such as those you are experiencing with health anxiety.

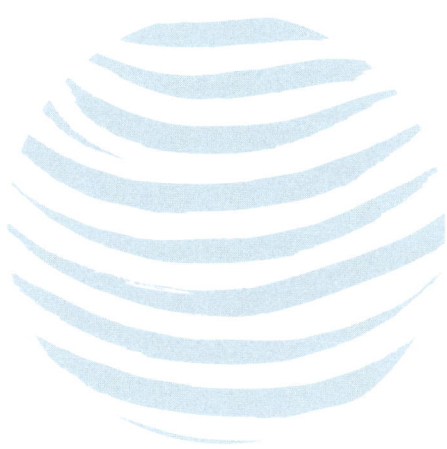

Pause and reflect

Now that you have worked your way through this book this far, use this page to pause and reflect on how you are feeling right now. You can do this freely or use these prompts below:

Describe what you are experiencing emotionally and physically, and write down any thoughts.

Note anything you have read in this book so far that has stayed with you. Repeating it here helps you to reinforce and remember it.

Jot down the things you have tried that helped you.

Hypnotherapy

In hypnotherapy, you're put into a deeply relaxed state by a hypnotherapist to change patterns of thoughts and behaviours through the power of positive suggestion. It's a myth that you're not in control of what's happening. It's a very common approach to managing all sorts of anxiety, including health anxiety and OCD. However, it isn't considered suitable if you have a history of psychosis.

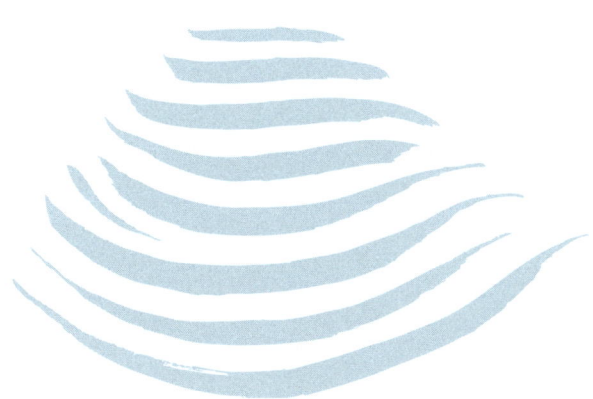

Bioenergetics analysis

The European Association for Psychotherapy describes bioenergetic analysis (BA) as a "psychotherapeutic method that pays attention to the bodily expressions such as gestures, mimics, voice and breathing patterns".

The term bioenergetics means dealing with the energy of life. It is rooted in psychoanalysis, but BA pays detailed attention to how your body expresses itself. It, like many therapies, considers the mind and body as one and the same, capable of impacting one another.

The concept of "character armouring" by Wilhelm Reich (where BA work was originally rooted) explains why emotionally traumatic experiences from childhood can cause certain muscular regions to tighten to protect themselves from further harm, impacting the ability to sense and feel. A core belief in bioenergetics (life energy) is that our bodies rely on energy sources to determine how we express our physical, emotional and spiritual selves.

Nature therapy

A review published in *Science Advances* in 2021 suggested that spending time in nature improves attitude, emotion and feelings. This can include the following:

- **Ecotherapy**: processing your feelings while doing outdoor activities in nature, such as hiking or gardening.
- **Nature-assisted therapy**: adopting a traditional talking therapy, but instead of being in a room, you're talking with your therapist outdoors. Some therapists offer "walk and talk" therapy, for example.
- **Wilderness therapy**: spending long periods of time in wild forests for activities such as survival skills training, boot camps or camping.
- **Green exercise**: taking an exercise class, such as aerobics, or doing a workout in a green space outdoors like the garden or a local park.

SHINRIN-YOKU FOREST BATHING

This is a Japanese technique of guided walks and mindful practice in forest settings. *Shinrin* in Japanese means forest – and *yoku* means bath. Through your senses, you connect your body to the natural world, helping you to go off-grid for a short while and slow down. This can be a great way to avoid spending too much screen time checking symptoms. It brings you into the present moment and de-stresses you.

To forest bathe effectively, switch off your phone and devices and take a walk without any goals or aims to get anywhere. Follow what your body wants to do and the direction it wants to take, savouring everything you see, hear and smell along the way.

Research shows that trees and plants emit phytoncides – aromatic compounds that trigger biological changes in the body when inhaled – in a similar way to aromatherapy, creating white blood cells that prevent illness. Studies have linked nature to anxiety symptom relief. For example, a 2015 study in *Proceedings of the National Academy of Sciences* found that people who walked for 90 minutes in a natural setting were less likely to ruminate than people who walked in an urban area.

It is also understood that the air near moving water, forests and mountains contains high levels of negative ions, which reduce the symptoms of depression that can often go along with health anxiety.

Reiki

Reiki is a Japanese technique that works by rebalancing "energy flow" over your body as a practitioner hovers their hands lightly above you. It can support the body to self-regulate and heal itself by unblocking pathways. This technique is performed while you are fully clothed and can bring about a tingly sensation.

For some people, benefits include lower stress levels and improved mood and sleep. Small amounts of research suggest that reiki has an impact on the autonomic nervous system, which regulates heart rate, blood pressure and breathing, as well as activating the parasympathetic nervous system and reducing cortisol levels. It's non-invasive and the risks are very low.

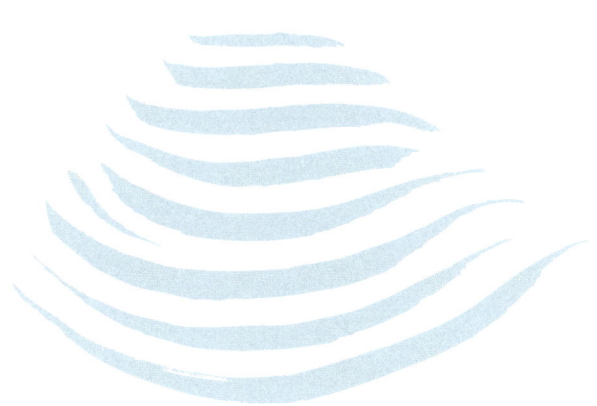

Meeting your anxiety

Put your anxiety in the room. Imagine it as a person. What does it look like; how does it approach you? If it came up to you at a party, how would you greet each other, and what would you make of it? Is it gendered? Older or younger? How are they dressed? Would you want a conversation with them? The idea here is that you are making friends with it or getting to know it a little better first rather than fighting it as soon as it appears. Write down your thoughts below.

Working with qi or meridian lines

In traditional Chinese medicine (TCM), there is the concept of the meridian system. Meridians are pathways in our body through which life-force energy flows. This vital energy is called *qi* (or *chi*), and optimum health is believed to be maintained when the flow of this energy is balanced and not blocked. Different emotional events in our lives can affect this flow and create blockages.

There are a number of different alternative therapies that operate from the concept of meridians and flow of *qi*, a few of which are described below.

ACUPUNCTURE

Acupuncture is a common form of TCM. It involves a highly skilled and trained acupuncturist inserting very fine needles into specific parts of your body. This encourages the movement of *qi* in your body by stimulating sensory nerves in the skin and muscles. It works well with meditation practices to calm the nervous system, which plays a huge role in reducing anxiety.

SHIATSU

Shiatsu is based on TCM, like acupuncture. However, the practitioner uses their hands and fingers on acupressure points or meridians, rather than needles. It is understood to reduce levels of cortisol — the stress hormone — in your body, lower your blood pressure and heart rate, increase the amount of the feel-good neurotransmitter serotonin, and increase oxytocin, which helps you to feel calm and relaxed.

In TCM, our mind and emotions cannot be separated from the body and each organ has an associated emotion and meridian. Your practitioner will work with the organs associated with fear and worry, which are your stomach and kidneys.

CUPPING

Cupping is practised across the world and, like acupuncture and shiatsu, works to restore the flow of *qi*. It involves applying a heated, round glass cup onto parts of the body that feel painful (often on the back). This creates a vacuum suction, which encourages blood flow to that area.

Other TCM techniques that work with *qi* flow include moxibustion (burning dry herbs), *tui na* massage (a mix of acupressure and massage) and Chinese herbal medicine.

Herbal remedies

Herbal remedies come from plants and can be in capsules, teas, drops or creams. They're usually available in most health stores or pharmacies, or you can visit a herbal practitioner. They are part of Ayurvedic and ancient Chinese medicine. Unlike psychiatric medication, these remedies can be tailor-made to your specific needs by the herbal practitioner, and you don't require a prescription. However, they can still cause side effects, so if that's a worry for you, it might be worth bearing in mind: herbal medicines affect the body, just like conventional medicines do. If you're taking other medication, herbal medicines can make these less effective. It is also worth knowing that tailor-made remedies aren't all licensed or subject to regulation. If you are very young, very old, pregnant or breastfeeding, take special care by speaking to your doctor first.

If you find yourself becoming more anxious as a result of thinking about all of these grey areas, try one of the other therapies listed in this book instead. You should always feel comfortable with what you are doing.

Let your brain flow

Pick up a pen and use this page to write whatever comes into your mind. Even if it's the same word repeated over and over for a few lines, let it arrive. Keep going until something starts to make sense. This can help free you up from the need to do things right and help you play around with making mistakes and a mess.

Weighted blankets

These are blankets lined with heavy materials, such as metal, which apply pressure on you while you sleep. They are very common for people with anxiety and health anxiety, especially if you're prone to panic, as they support a feeling of containment and grounding and mimic the effect of a hug or tight swaddling on newborns. The blankets are very safe, but you might not like them if you get claustrophobic. Studies into how effective weighted blankets are for reducing anxiety have mixed results but, anecdotally, they are reported to be particularly supportive for neurodivergent people. Anxiety is a significant issue for neurodivergent children. A qualitative study exploring parental experiences of their children's behaviour following the use of a weighted blanket when going to sleep suggests that weighted blankets contribute to reduced anxiety in children with attention deficit hyperactivity disorder (ADHD), resulting in a better night's sleep and improved mastery over life during waking hours.

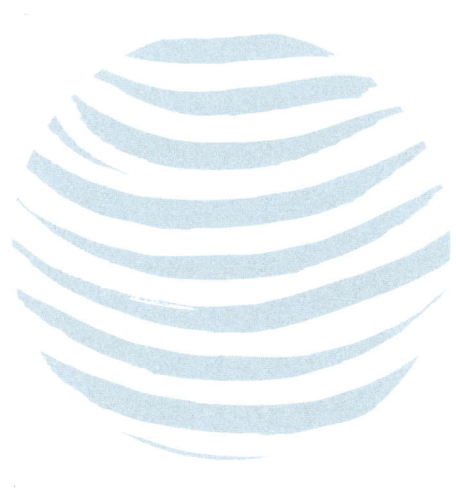

Get dancing

Dance is part of most cultures worldwide, enjoyed socially or as an art form. Dance movement psychotherapy (DMP) is an established practice used in many clinical settings. The Association for Dance Movement Psychotherapy in the UK describes DMP as a therapy that recognizes how body movement is a form of communication and expression, like an instrument already hard-wired into us. It sees strong links between emotion and movement and can help you increase self-awareness and develop tools for managing overwhelming feelings. But dance doesn't just have to happen in therapy: the beauty of it is that you can dance anywhere, anytime, on your own or with others, as part of a class, on the dancefloor at a club or wedding, or in your own bedroom. Along with the usual benefits of cardiovascular exercise — muscle strength, improved posture and increased flexibility — dancing helps you express your feelings. Below and on the following pages are some dance variations that may be helpful for health anxiety.

5RHYTHMS

5Rhythms dance is a movement meditation practice drawing on a range of traditions, including shamanistic, mystical and Eastern philosophy. It usually takes place in groups in a class, where instructors play music and guide you. You move as you like, expressing and embodying your feelings.

HIP HOP

Hip hop dance includes a range of street dancing and is usually performed in outdoor spaces or through dance classes. Dances are improvised. There is extensive research showing that the culture of hip hop, through the combination of words and physical body movement, is healing for mental health issues such as anxiety.

ECSTATIC DANCE

Also referred to as conscious dance, this encourages you to use unchoreographed movements to discover yourself. A recent University of California health study showed that ecstatic dance improved the well-being of participants with anxiety and a history of trauma.

BELLY DANCE

Belly dance is a Middle Eastern and North African dance art rooted in Egypt, though there are variations around the world. It is suitable for any age, gender and body type. The connection to the body through sensual movement can be very grounding. With health anxiety, it is possible to be hyper-focused on certain parts of the body while disconnected to the body as a whole. Through learning to master techniques that manipulate body parts, we can reaffirm a feeling of mastery and control over the body, which can be increased with practice. Depending on where you are in the world, you might learn the dance in a studio class or in a community group, or you might have a personal teacher who guides you. It is a culturally sensitive dance form, so it is wise to learn the movements and how they relate to Arabic beats and lyrics from a teacher with a strong understanding of the culture. If you were raised within Arabic, Middle Eastern or North African culture, then the dance will likely already be a familiar part of social gatherings, weddings and cultural events.

Formal dance

Styles such as ballet, tap, jazz, ballroom and Latin are more structured and require practice, but the routine and discipline of this can be helpful in supporting you to shift your focus away from intrusive thoughts. You usually learn alongside the same cohort of people in your group through weekly classes and work your way up through grades, or you can go to classes as you wish.

These sessions usually lead to opportunities to meet people, make friends and find community through social events, dance clubs, competitions and performances. This is important when you are feeling isolated through anxiety. Many of these dances require careful footwork and contact with the floor, which links right back to grounding, so it can be a helpful practice to get into. If you are not too keen on learning a dance style but wish to incorporate dance movement into your exercise routine, then aerobic classes such as Zumba are a fun and more freeing option. Remembering what step needs to come next is part of creating new neural pathways and rechannelling thoughts.

Acting out

Psychodrama can help increase spontaneity. It is an experiential approach to therapy that involves role-playing. The fill-in pages on page 139 and 140 will play on this idea and give you tips for how to incorporate psychodrama in your life. Joseph Moreno, the founder of psychodrama, recognized that anxiety decreases spontaneity, and the same applies the other way around. As such, the more you can get used to improvisation and role-playing, the more your anxiety diminishes.

It isn't about being impulsive but freeing yourself up to feel alive. Psychodrama addresses anxiety in several ways. It helps to close the door on unresolved issues connected to your health anxiety, for example, if the anxiety was triggered through a real experience of witnessing someone being ill or some other trauma. It also helps you act out future situations to deal with future fears. This is a playful approach that can increase your confidence and trust in yourself. You will already have experienced some of these in this book.

Top Dog/Underdog

If you find yourself repeating the phrase "yes, but" after being given reassurance, it may be because the part of you that is full of doubt is overpowering everything else. In these moments, a technique called Top Dog/Underdog can be helpful. This technique describes the anxious relationship people have with themselves. The "Top Dog" is the part of a person who demands they meet certain standards, and the "Underdog" resists, making excuses as to why these demands are not met.

Underneath the "Underdog" column on the next page, write all the statements you can think of that are meant to be reassuring — like mantras you repeat to yourself when you are trying to cope, or ideas that other people have put to you. These include statements mentioned in this book. In the "Top Dog" column, write down the counterargument.

At the end of this exercise, you should have a list of supportive statements and another list of reasons why your Top Dog isn't convinced that they are true. This raises your awareness and insight into what the two parts of you are saying.

Underdog	Top Dog

Top Dog/Underdog 2: Making friends

Take a look at the Top Dog/Underdog exercise you did on the previous page. Notice how the voices in both columns are having a fight. One is always trying to win over the other. When life feels okay, you probably notice the reassuring Underdog winning out while, at other times, the doubting Top Dog is overpowering. The energy you spend on this fight can be exhausting.

Instead of having them fight, get them to become friends. How will they do that? Write your ideas down here.

....

....

....

....

....

....

....

....

....

....

Top Dog/Underdog 3: Confront it

You could call this the "What do you want from me?" technique.

What is it your two voices want from each other? If you were to imagine these two voices stopping for a moment to discuss what it is they want the other to understand, what would it be? This exercise can be helpful to understand what is driving this fight.

Some other questions to ask:

"What do you want from me?"

"What's in it for you if I do what you say?"

"What does it matter to you that I don't do what you want?"

"Why do you care what I do?"

"Do you trust me to know what to do myself?"

"Can you help me?"

Top Dog/Underdog 4: Shift position

To elaborate on the previous exercise, place two chairs in the room: one representing your Underdog and the other the Top Dog. Physically switch from one chair to the other, talking from each perspective, and see what emerges. Moving from chair to chair in this way can sometimes help you to completely embody one side of the argument over the other.

Top Dog/Underdog 5: Voice it

Go back to your original column on page 139. Who do these voices remind you of?

Sometimes, when you examine the quality of the voices and how the two speak to each other, it can remind you of a relationship dynamic you already have: that might be with your parents, a partner, teachers or a boss. What is it you want from those people when you get into those sorts of conversations? That might give you a clue for how these two voices can now help each other.

Supporting someone

Seeing someone you care about struggle is never easy. Perhaps you've noticed a change in their behaviour that worries you, or you can see that their anxiety is affecting their life. It can be easy to feel responsible or go above and beyond what we feel we are capable of managing, but try to avoid acting out of guilt. This can lead to burnout. The next few pages will arm you with tips for how to manage this situation.

CHANGE YOUR MINDSET

A person living with health anxiety will likely feel a lot of shame. They know that what is happening doesn't feel rational, but their brain is doing something they don't know how to stop. They feel like an open tap that's stuck. The experience can feel confusing and scary, and sometimes the biggest help is simply being able to hear what it's like for them – without you needing to know what to do about it. People with health anxiety often report that if they knew what to do to make it stop, they would.

CHECK IN

This doesn't have to mean spending long periods of time with them unless you want it to. It's okay if you don't have the time to talk. A quick text message to let them know they're on your mind, a letter in the post or a short phone call on the way to work can all help. Simply letting them know you're around can be enough. This can be helpful when you don't know what to say to help, but you want them to know you care.

DON'T OVERPROMISE

Instead of: "Call me anytime."
Try: "I've got a few minutes in my lunch break to give you a call."

BE CLEAR AND SPECIFIC

You could say: "I'm going to be out of contact for a few days because I'm going away, but I could pop round for half an hour in the evening."

DON'T RETREAT

You might start to feel like you want to distance yourself or avoid the situation. It's understandable. But there is something you can do.

CREATE BOUNDARIES

The knock-on effect of supporting someone else can take its toll. Boundaries keep everybody involved safe, and they are used in therapy for a reason. If you picture a tall building and imagine yourself standing on top of it, you are unlikely to want to go close to the edge if there are no railings. But when you create a strong fence around the periphery, it supports you to feel safer and to approach and lean in.

WHAT TO DO AND SAY

If someone opens up to you, respect their privacy and always assume that what they tell you is confidential unless they let you know otherwise. You should also do the following:

- Give them space.
- Don't rush to respond.
- Reflect back what you're hearing them say.
- Be clear about what they need from you: is it a hug, a listening ear, advice, an answer? A helpful statement might be: "I'm good at listening, is that what you need or is it something else?" Or: "I've been through this before and have some advice I can offer based on my own experience. Do you want that?"
- Avoid giving your opinion or judgement.
- Hold back on advice.
- Focus on feelings, not what happened.

- Ask open-ended questions. These are questions that invite more and don't lead to a "yes" or "no" answer. For example, instead of: "Are you feeling panicky?" Try: "What are you feeling?"

It can be tempting to want to offer solutions, but try not to unless that's what they've come to you for.

Be prepared to offer something else. You might offer to take them out or distract them in some other way. It's worth checking with them now and again to see what kind of support they usually find more useful when they're with you.

TAKE THE PRESSURE OFF

Remember that you're not a therapist: you won't get everything right. Therapists have spent years training in how to listen and provide support, so lower your expectations of yourself. The best you can do is good enough. If you're feeling pressured into giving more than you can, be as honest as possible about your limitations and signpost them elsewhere. That might start with simply giving them this book. And don't forget to factor in your own self-care: take time out for yourself and make use of the resources in this book.

Remember this: you did not cause their health anxiety and you won't be the one to fix it either. What you can be is encouraging.

Be internet savvy

If talking to anyone directly feels too much right now, there are online options to support you.

The internet can be a murky place, but there are some carefully vetted online peer-to-peer forums you can access that are monitored. If you are aged 16–24, TalkLife is a carefully regulated forum for young people to explore any issue in confidence. You can also contribute blogs and articles to the site.

Social media can be a quick way to find like-minded people in a similar situation. Many social media platforms, such as X (formerly known as Twitter), have a hashtag function that is useful on anxiety awareness days, when charities will usually encourage anybody struggling to connect using the hashtag. The TalkCampus app also offers mental health support for more than 80 universities worldwide across 26 languages.

Remember that social media is public. Never post anything that you aren't comfortable being out there. When online, be wary of pop-up adverts and flashing logos from individuals or profit-making companies offering support – many algorithms are alert to Google searches and take advantage. Always take time to research organizations and use the resources section in this book. Be especially careful with community forums and social media, even in private groups. It's easy to air your thoughts online, but posts can be retweeted, screenshotted and shared. These spaces are subject to trolling, harmful advice and misinformation.

When nothing works

If you have arrived here and do not feel like you have got the answers you need, try not to feel disheartened or lose hope. Everyone's pace is different and there will be others in the same boat. The back of this book is packed full of resources to signpost you forwards, but the crucial thing to do is stay connected and keep up your support.

If things feel so bad that you feel in crisis or are having suicidal thoughts, don't fight this alone. In an emergency, you have options to contact a crisis team, visit a crisis house, go directly to hospital or call a crisis helpline.

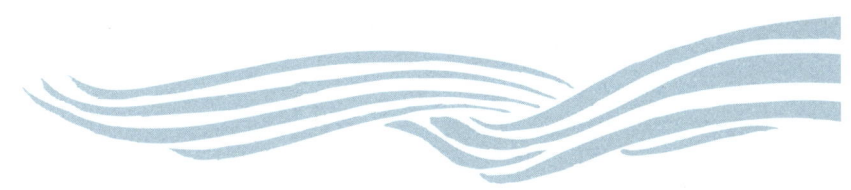

Conclusion

You should now have a clearer understanding of what health anxiety is, the science behind it, and how to spot the signs and triggers. You have seen tips for how to support yourself to cope, as well as who and where to go to if you need more structured or formal help.

If you have health anxiety or you are supporting someone with health anxiety, this book will hopefully go some way to helping you understand what's going on for you or the person in your life and give you tools to cope. Whether you were already far into your journey with health anxiety before picking up this book or you were feeling out of sorts, unclear what it was and unsure of where to turn, you will have hopefully found something within these pages that feels grounding and supportive.

Feeling heard and understood is so important to recovery, and you deserve the right kind of support around you — whether that's friends, professionals or books, such as this one. Keep it safe to return to at any time you need it. Remind yourself, whoever you are and whichever stage you're at, you've got this. Good luck.

Resources

PROFESSIONAL BODIES

American Counseling Association: www.counseling.org
United Kingdom Council for Psychotherapy: www.psychotherapy.org.uk
British Association for Counselling and Psychotherapy: www.bacp.co.uk
British Psychological Society: www.bps.org.uk
Health & Care Professions Council: www.hcpc-uk.org

FOR COMPLEMENTARY AND ALTERNATIVE MEDICINE

In the UK: **Complementary and Natural Healthcare Council (CNHC)**: www.cnhc.org.uk

In the US: **The National Center for Complementary and Integrative Health (NCCIH)**: www.nccih.nih.gov

Worldwide: www.who.int/health-topics/traditional-complementary-and-integrative-medicine

Details on confidentiality: www.goodtherapy.org/blog/psychpedia/client-confidentiality

MENTAL HEALTH HELPLINES GLOBALLY

Befrienders Worldwide: www.befrienders.org
Crisis helplines: www.helpguide.org/find-help.htm
For a list of worldwide suicide helplines: www.suicidestop.com/call_a_hotline.html

THERAPY DIRECTORIES

Pink Therapy, supporting LGBTQ+: www.pinktherapy.com
College of Sexual and Relationship Therapists (CORST), for psychosexual and relationship therapists: www.cosrt.org.uk
Cruse, for bereavement: www.cruse.org.uk
International Therapist Directory: www.internationaltherapistdirectory.com/all-locations/
Psychiatric medication: www.mind.org.uk/information-support/drugs-and-treatments/medication/drug-names-a-z/
EMDR International Association (EMDRIA): www.emdria.org/about-emdr-therapy/

BOOKS

Eleanor Morgan, *Anxiety for Beginners* (2016)
Natasha Devon, *A Beginner's Guide to Being Mental* (2018)
Ariane Sherine, *Talk Yourself Better* (2018)
Tim Grayburn, *Boys Don't Cry* (2018)

PODCASTS

Mental – The Podcast to Destigmatise Mental Health hosted by Bobby Temps: Breaking down mental health stigma and discrimination through honest mental health interviews.
Bryony Gordon's Mad World: Intimate conversations about getting unwell – and getting better.
The Anxiety Coaches Podcast hosted by Gina Ryan: Inspiring conversations sharing lifestyle changes to calm your nervous system and help you heal anxiety, panic, stress and post-traumatic stress disorder (PTSD).

UK CHARITIES

Anxiety UK: www.anxietyuk.org.uk

Campaign Against Living Miserably (CALM): www.thecalmzone.net/

Combat Stress for Veteran's Mental Health: www.combatstress.org.uk

Mental Health Foundation: www.mentalhealth.org.uk

MIND: mind.org.uk

Samaritans: www.samaritans.org, call 116 123 or email jo@samaritans.org

List of charities across the UK: www.wheretotalk.org/charities/

If you're sectioned in the UK – Royal College of Psychiatrists: www.rcpsych.ac.uk/mental-health/treatments-and-wellbeing/beingsectioned?searchTerms=being%20sectioned

Self-referral through the NHS Talking Therapies service: www.nhs.uk/service-search/mental-health/find-an-nhs-talking-therapies-service

US CHARITIES

National Alliance on Mental Illness (NAMI): www.nami.org

To Write Love On Her Arms: Depression, Addiction, Self-injury and Suicide: www.twloha.com/

If you're committed in the US — Treatment Advocacy Center: www.treatmentadvocacycenter.org/

WORLDWIDE

Brain and Behavior Research Foundation: bbrfoundation.org/

The Jed Foundation, teen and young adult suicide prevention: jedfoundation.org/

Rethink: rethink.org/

StrongMinds: Treating depression in Africa for women and young people: strongminds.org/

TalkLife: talklife.com

About the Author

Katy Georgiou is a practising clinical supervisor and gestalt psychotherapist accredited with the UKCP and BACP. She works in private practice and within a GP surgery counselling service. She also works with the British Association for Performing Arts Medicine and Music Minds Matter delivering therapy, workshops and support groups to music industry professionals. She is the founder, host and producer of Sound Affects Podcast – a music and mental health podcast featured in *NME*, *Psychologies* and *Therapy Today*. She regularly features in the media and on panels on issues around therapy and mental health, including BBC Radio, and has authored two previous books on the subject. She edits the Ethical Dilemmas section of *Therapy Today* magazine. An experienced journalist, Katy has written for *The Times*, *The Guardian*, *The Independent*, *Newsweek*, Metro and *Psychologies*, among others. She is also a former Samaritans helpline listener and has worked in NHS psychiatric hospitals and in HM government prisons.

Previous books by Katy:
How to Understand and Deal with Stress
Your Mind Matters: How to Talk about Your Mental Health

Website: www.kgcounsellor.com
Twitter/X: @kgcounsellor

Notes

How to Understand and Deal with Anxiety

Everything You Need to Know to Manage Anxiety

RASHA BARRAGE
978-1-80007-425-5

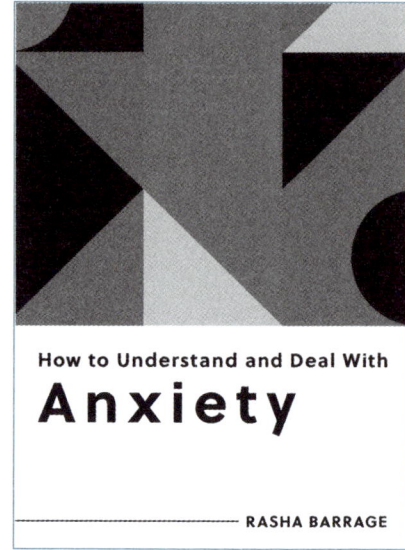

How to Understand and Deal with Depression

Everything You Need to Know to Manage Depression

WENDY GREEN
978-1-80007-426-2

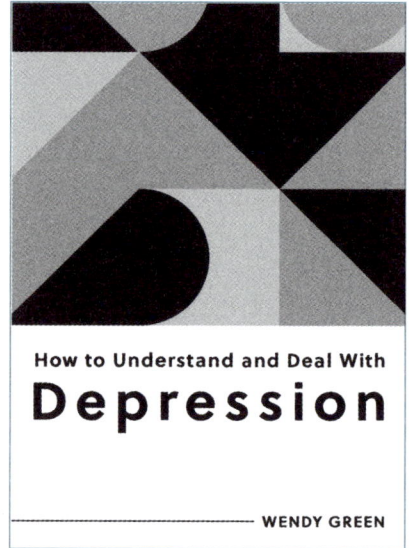

How to Understand and Deal with Social Anxiety

Everything You Need to Know to Manage Social Anxiety

MITA MISTRY

978-1-80007-496-5

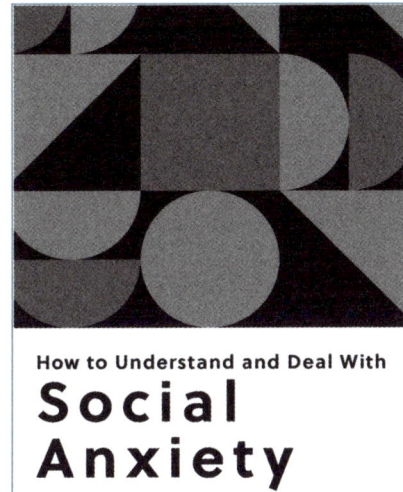

How to Understand and Deal With
Social Anxiety

———————————————— MITA MISTRY

How to Understand and Deal with Stress

Everything You Need to Know to Manage Stress

KATY GEORGIOU

978-1-80007-424-8

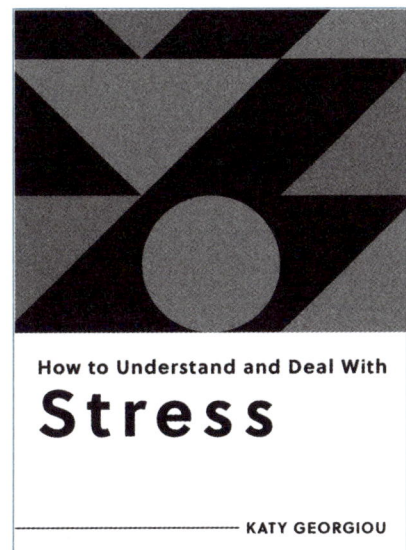

How to Understand and Deal With
Stress

———————————————— KATY GEORGIOU

Have you enjoyed this book?

If so, why not write a review on your favourite website?

If you're interested in finding out more about our books,
find us on Facebook at Summersdale Publishers,
on Twitter/X at @Summersdale and on Instagram and
TikTok at @summersdalebooks and get in touch.
We'd love to hear from you!

Thanks very much for buying this Summersdale book.

www.summersdale.com